Practical Medical Ethics

David Seedhouse
The University of Liverpool, UK

and

Lisetta Lovett
Consultant in Psychiatry
St George's Hospital
Stafford, UK

JOHN WILEY & SONS
Chichester · New York · Brisbane · Toronto · Singapore

Other Wiley Editorial Offices

John Wiley & Sons, Inc., 605 Third Avenue,
New York, NY 10158-0012, USA

Jacaranda Wiley Ltd, G.P.O. Box 859, Brisbane,
Queensland 4001, Australia

John Wiley & Sons (Canada) Ltd, 22 Worcester Road,
Rexdale, Ontario M9W 1L1, Canada

John Wiley & Sons (SEA) Pte Ltd, 37 Jalan Pemimpin #05-04,
Block B, Union Industrial Building, Singapore 2057

Library of Congress Cataloging-in-Publication Data

Seedhouse, David.
    Practical medical ethics / David Seedhouse, Lisetta Lovett.
        p. cm.
    Includes bibliographical references and index.
    ISBN 0 471 92843 7
    1. Medical ethics. I. Lovett, Lisetta. II. Title.
    [DNLM: 1. Ethics, Medical. W 50 S451p]
    R724.S434 1992
    174'.2—dc20
    DNLM/DLC
    for Library of Congress   91-27614
                                                                  CIP

British Library Cataloguing in Publication Data

A catalogue record for this book is
available from the British Library

ISBN 0471 92843 7

Typeset in Times 10/12 pt by Photo·graphics, Honiton, Devon
Printed in Great Britain by BAS Printers Limited, Over Wallop, Hampshire

Contents

Acknowledgements

We would like to thank the following people for their comments and advice:

Dr David Chadwick, Consultant Neurologist, Walton Hospital

Dr Nick Davies, Research Registrar, Department of Surgery, University of Liverpool

Dr Chris Dowrick, Lecturer, Department of General Practice, University of Liverpool

Dr David Glasgow, Lecturer, Department of Clinical Psychology, University of Liverpool

Dr Jonathan Lovett, Consultant Child & Adolescent Psychiatrist, Family Counselling Service, Crewe

We also thank Elizabeth Fearon for her patience and persistence with the typing of the numerous drafts which this book required

Lisetta Lovett wishes to extend special thanks to her husband Jonathan for his support whilst working on the text at Bird Island

Introduction

The Aims of this Book

This book is designed to introduce medical students and practising doctors to the function of ethics in medical work. The book aims specifically:

> To present a range of problems drawn from medical practice which can best be solved from a base in ethical theory;
>
> To teach practical decision-making methods in order to enable doctors to engage in independent ethical analysis.

The book concentrates on areas of medical activity where decision making is particularly ethically complex, and provides an accessible 'way in' to philosophical analysis for clinicians. By explaining two practical problem-solving instruments rooted in ethical theory, and by demonstrating how each might be applied over a variety of cases, it is envisaged that teachers and students will gain sufficient expertise to work independently. Naturally, in a short teaching guide book only a few examples can be discussed, but each has been carefully selected so as to have general relevance as well as specific interest.

When trying out the decision-making guides the reader must bear in mind that both contain certain assumptions about the nature of ethics and moral reasoning which are not universally held.* In order not to mislead, these assumptions are explained in this introduction.

The authors aim to avoid:

> Providing a comprehensive theoretical account of the role of ethical analysis in medicine;
>
> Offering simplistic solutions to inherently complex problems;
>
> Presenting a dogmatic point of view;
>
> Clouding the meaning of common English with unnecessary jargon.

---

* It should also be noted that some of the analyses contained within the book do not reflect the opinions of the authors.

The analyses offered are not as precisely dissected as they would be in a purely philosophical text. However, the point of the book is not to engage in the finer points of technical philosophy, but to show that ethical analysis is a skill which can be learnt – just like all other clinical skills.

Why Should Doctors Study Ethics?

The nature of ethics in medicine is often misunderstood. In order to appreciate the importance of ethical analysis to clinical work it is first necessary to dispel some illusions. Two beliefs in particular, both of them false, continue to be widely held.

One common misperception is that ethics and medicine are independent subjects and that when they do come into contact then ethics is merely an adjunct to medical activity. The general consensus amongst clinicians still seems to be that doctors should provide the finest possible clinical care, and *in addition* ought to have high ethical standards.

A further false belief is often encountered in medicine. It is that these 'high ethical standards' can be discovered in Codes, Oaths and Declarations. Such is the influence of this myth that several British universities encourage medical graduands to swear the Declaration of Geneva or the Hippocratic Oath. As a result the error is perpetuated, and these primitive codes of practice continue to receive an unwarranted reverence. Dependent on his university, the embryonic doctor will make such statements as:

> 'I will respect the secrets which are confided in me, even after the patient has died'[1]

or

> 'I will give no deadly medicine to anyone if asked, nor suggest any such counsel; and in like manner I will not give a woman a pessary to produce abortion. With purity and holiness I will pass my life and practise my art.'[2]

Few house officers need to reflect upon their practical problems of care for long to understand that these are inadequate rules. Even if a graduate finds that he agrees with them he will soon learn that there are equally forceful alternatives which he must consider, and for which his colleagues can make powerful cases.

This casebook establishes that ethics is irrevocably linked to the practice of medicine, and that a far more comprehensive and flexible method of making decisions is needed by doctors. Ethical 'commandments', however imposing they might seem, and however much they are steeped in history, are simply not enough.

---

1. Declaration of Geneva.
2. Hippocratic Oath.

A False Picture of Ethics in Medicine

It is a major error to picture 'ethics' and 'medicine' as if they were two separate boxes like this:

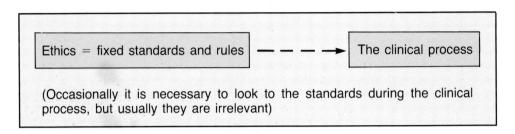

Fig. 1 A false picture of ethics in medicine

Four fallacies

The creed that ethics is a peripheral subject to which doctors need refer only in special circumstances depends on four specific fallacies. These are:

1. That it is possible to make a clear distinction between 'clinical analysis' and 'ethical analysis' in health care;

2. That 'professional ethics' is a different category of thinking to 'the ethics of daily life';

3. That there is a body of relatively uncontroversial 'ethical standards';

4. That ethics in medicine is ultimately 'just a matter of opinion'.

These are pervasive beliefs, but their popularity does not make them any the less fallacious. Brief reflection on an actual medical situation will serve to show their weaknesses:

Doctor X is considering whether or not to break a confidence. A patient has presented with a sexually transmitted infection which he wishes to have treated without anyone else knowing that he has it. Not even his wife is to know. On questioning it becomes obvious to the doctor that the wife, who is also a patient, is likely to have the infection, probably does not yet realise it, and would certainly benefit from the speediest medical attention.

What should Doctor X do?

The doctor must make a decision. If the four fallacies were truths it would be relatively easy for him to decide – he would need only to consult the appropriate professional guidelines and announce his opinion. However there is no single *right answer*, rather there are a number of *possible policies*, all of which can seem justifiable to some degree.

Basic options for Doctor X Doctor X might simply say nothing, and wait until the wife presents with an infection – so maintaining confidentiality (in line with most Oaths). Still keeping the secret he might collude with the husband and call the wife in, perhaps for a screening service – so facilitating early treatment whilst not abusing the husband's trust. Alternatively, he might decide that this is an issue which the husband and wife must talk about, and so find some way of seeing the couple together. Or he might form the opinion that he has a duty to tell the wife about her disease, and that this duty must take precedence over any 'duty to keep confidences'.

Each course of action has drawbacks. If Doctor X says nothing and waits then the wife may be caused unnecessary physical suffering in addition to a natural anxiety as the condition becomes manifest. If he colludes with the husband he then becomes embroiled in a deceit in which he respects the wishes of one of his patients whilst concealing the truth from the other. If he attempts to bring the husband and wife together to work out the problem he runs the risk of alienating them both, and of being the catalyst of a marital crisis. And if Doctor X chooses to break the confidence outright he is again likely to stoke trouble in the relationship, on top of which it is probable that he will lose the trust of the man forever.

Addressing the Fallacies

Against fallacy 1: Clinical and ethical analysis in health care are inseparable

The above example is one of an indefinite number which show that *clinical analysis* and *ethical analysis* in health work are inextricably linked. Any attempt to separate out the two processes can be done only theoretically. In reality the 'two processes' make sense only when seen together. Only by the construction of hypothetical models do they appear to be activities of different kinds. In any situation where his task is to work for the health of a person a clinician must draw on *both* clinical and ethical theory, and he must make use of them in tandem. He must ask '*clinical questions*': 'what is this condition?', 'what is the best treatment for it?', and 'how might the therapeutic programme best be managed?'. But these questions are meaningful in human terms only if placed within the context of '*ethical questions*': 'what should my role be in this intervention?', 'what duties do I have?', 'what is the preferred outcome?', and 'to what extent should I respect the wishes of my patient?' Whether the issue is how much information to give, how much time to spend, whether to be authoritative, whether to share doubt, or which medical option to take, it is never the case that the deliberation can be purely clinical, as if made in laboratory conditions. Other factors such as the beliefs held by patients about therapies, the financial costs of treatment, and the impact of any medical intervention on others are essential considerations. Ethical analysis takes these and many other factors into account and so is an indispensable part of clinical work.

The necessary connection of ethical analysis and clinical analysis: a further example Consider the doctor who has a brief to work for public health. Naturally he must decide which projects to devote his time to. Only the most inadequately educated doctor will base his decision entirely on precedent, or completely on the preferences of others. At some point, even if he is not entirely aware of the complexity of the intellectual process he is undertaking, he must think over his values and priorities. Should he, for instance, choose to work on projects which will concentrate resources on the whole community rather than a select few? Or should he target particularly deprived groups for special attention? In specific practical terms, should he strive for open access leisure facilities for all, or should he develop a project on 'budgeting for nutrition', so choosing to help only mothers shown to be most at risk of producing underweight babies?

In order to make a decision the doctor must involve himself in two basic levels of analysis:

The doctor asks:

Which public health project should I start?

In part his answer must be influenced by:

A. *Matters of Fact*

    1. His personal interests and preferences

    2. His contract of employment

    3. Government priorities

    4. Sources of funding

    5. Contemporary priorities of the medical culture

And, because the doctor is not governed solely by pragmatics:

B. *Matters of Principle*

    1. Philosophical foundations, such as theories of:
    Social justice
    Equality
    Need
    Moral rights

continued

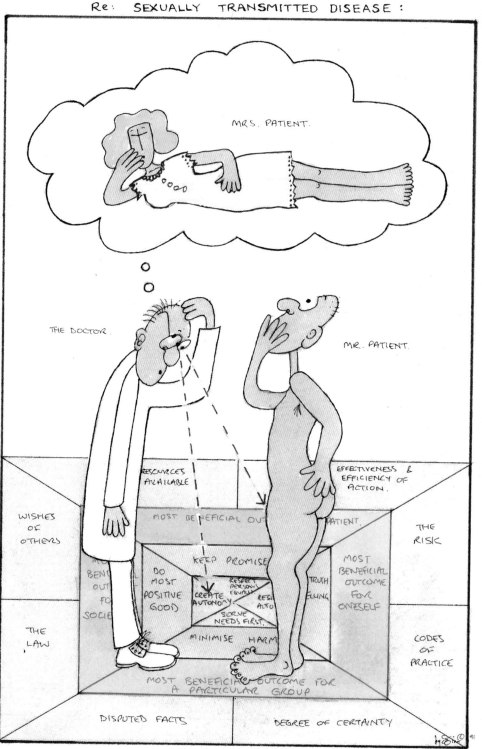

continued

> 2. The rationale of his work: *to what ultimate theoretical end is he striving?* (For instance, is his mission to increase social well-being, or to eradicate diseases, or some combination of these goals?)

Even if the doctor is acting purely on instructions, his superiors must, at some point, have reflected on theoretical principles, interpreted them and ranked them in order of perceived importance. No doctor can escape the influence of ethical theory and analysis.

Against fallacy 2: 'Professional ethics' and 'the ethics of daily life' are not radically different

When considering how he ought to intervene in other people's lives the professional is *essentially* in the same position as the 'lay-person'. In medical work some facts may be complicated and require a technical interpretation or a clinical skill may be needed in order to resolve a troublesome situation, but each and every problem of human intervention must be settled through a process of ethical analysis (moral deliberation), however specialised the technical requirements. Whether done by a 'professional' or a 'lay-person' (and we are all lay-people when not at work), the process involves balancing principles and theories against various precedents, opinions and facts before a decision is made.

For Doctor X there are technical questions about the best treatment for the clinical condition (as there will always be in medical cases), and there are general issues about how best to assist his fellow human beings. Equally, there are general questions facing the male patient. Some of these are identical to those which confront Doctor X: 'Should I tell the truth?' 'Should I collude?' 'Should I attempt to solve this problem single-handed?'. Although their starting points are different, both doctor and patient must go through a broadly similar deliberative process. The only significant differences are practical (the doctor does not have the disease, and he does have specialist knowledge), but these are outweighed by the commonalities.

Against fallacy 3: There are no uncontroversial 'ethical standards'

It is often said that four principles are basic to ethics in medicine: *beneficence, non-maleficence, justice* and *respect for autonomy*.[3] In everyday language the four principles mean 'do the most positive good' (*beneficence*), 'do no harm' (*non-maleficence*), 'be fair' (*justice*), and 'respect people's wishes' (*respect for autonomy*). However, even though they are accepted by a certain group of people, each principle can be interpreted in several different ways. This ambiguity raises a

---

3. *Journal of Medical Ethics*. London: IME Publications: *passim*.

more fundamental question about the standing of the principles themselves: are they truly the 'bed-rock' of ethics?

'Justice': an uncontroversial standard? Generally speaking most people wish to see 'fair play', especially where their personal affairs are concerned. None of us reacts well when we perceive that we are being treated 'unjustly'. If a person is working hard at his job, and yet his boss chooses to promote a lazy, less effective person over his head, then there will be an instinctive response that the boss is being 'unfair'. Such commonly held human feelings help create an illusion that justice is a simple principle which everyone understands in the same way.

However, when the 'principle of justice' is considered more dispassionately, at a theoretical level removed from personal perceptions of fairness, then it becomes far harder to say definitely what 'being fair' means. In philosophical writings justice has been understood in several ways, not all of which are compatible either in theory or when it comes to the implementation of 'just' policies in practice.

In health care the notion of 'justice' has come to have an especial significance in the context of *resource allocation*. No health care resource is infinitely available, and many (for example, donor organs) are in short supply. Given this scarcity of resources it is inevitable that questions arise about how best to allocate them, about how to ensure the fairest allocation of scarce benefits.

There are at least three alternative conceptions of justice. Each alternative is genuinely held by substantial numbers of people, yet each can produce different practical decisions about allocation. Followers of each conception claim theirs to be the most *basic* meaning of justice. The options are:

(a) To be just one should respect a person's *rights*.
[On this view of justice what matters most is to discover which people have legal or moral rights to desirable goods (for instance, to medical treatment), and then to ensure that these people receive what is due to them.]

(b) To be just one should reward a person according to what he *deserves*.
[On this view of justice what matters most is to discover which people have the most merit (for instance, which have the most talent, which have worked hardest, which have been most successful) and then to ensure that these people are rewarded in relation to what they deserve. In medicine this might mean that the most deserving ought to receive treatment before the less meritorious.]

(c) To be just one should reward a person according to what he *needs*.
[On this view of justice what matters most is to discover which people have the greatest need of a particular resource, and then to ensure that those people (for instance, the poorest, the sickest, or the weakest) receive it.]

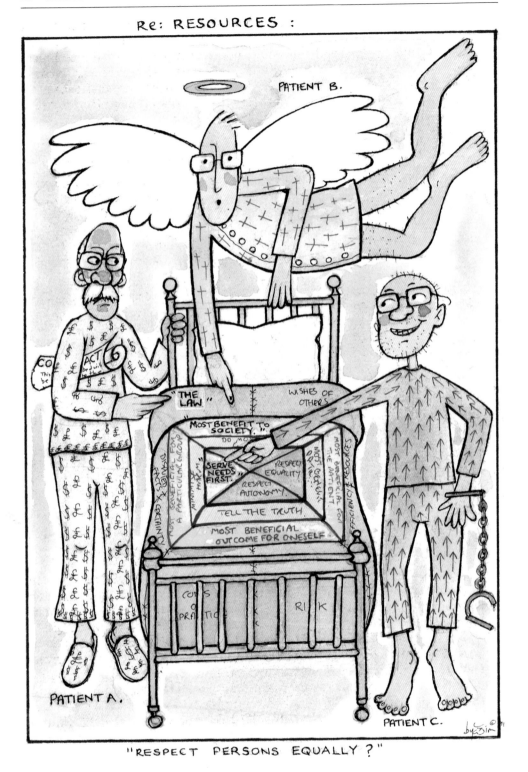

Each secondary 'principle' within the 'principle of justice' can be in competition with the others – so which should we regard as basic? To address *this* question properly it would be necessary to enter the technical realm of social and political philosophy in some detail. However, the purpose here is merely to demonstrate that it is a fallacy to believe that there can be uncontroversial ethical standards. For this it is necessary only to use a simple example:

Doctor Y has only one bed remaining on his ward, and three people whom he might help. It is up to the doctor to choose whether or not to treat a private patient or a patient under the NHS insurance scheme. (*Note: Assume this choice exists, and that there is no alternative way forward.*) Each of the potential patients A, B and C are candidates for a cataract operation but each has different circumstances.

Potential Patient A is Doctor Y's private patient who has recently inherited the family business. He has a contract with the doctor which guarantees him most medical treatment, including this treatment, as appropriate. Thus Patient A has a specific contractual right to treatment. However, Patient A has 'reasonable vision' and could work for at least another year.

Potential Patient B is an NHS patient and an extremely hardworking employee of a charitable organisation. He works with the homeless and receives only minimal wages. He now has difficulty with his vision, but could continue to work for six months more.

Potential Patient C is also an NHS patient. He has a long criminal record for breaking and entering, and is currently unemployed. He prides himself on never having worked for anything in his life, and he sees no reason to start now. Patient C is virtually blind and may become permanently blind unless he is operated on very soon.

The question is this: how can the doctor who would be *just* choose between the three potential patients? If he believes that justice is basically a question of distributing benefit according to a person's *rights* then he might favour Potential Patient A since this patient has an explicit contract (giving him a legal right). Alternatively, if he feels that justice is essentially a matter of rewarding people on *merit* he might choose to offer the bed to Potential Patient B. However, if he is of the opinion that the truest sense of justice is to help those with greatest *need* first then he may well prefer Potential Patient C.

Even such a basic scenario becomes very complicated on analysis. But at least one thing is clear: it is no answer to the problem for the doctor merely to say 'I propose to be just'.

Single principles are not enough   Solutions to 'ethical problems' cannot be had merely by selecting a particular principle and simply asserting that 'this is the answer'. Even cursory thought about Doctor X's dilemma shows the naivety of this belief. Choosing principles habitually, or in rote fashion, to solve complex problems of life is obviously an inadequate strategy. Any doctor who adopts such a policy can expect little respect from either her colleagues or her patients.

To give a further brief example: if, as is quite often the case, two people disagree about what counts as a harm (or what counts as the most significant harm) then the meaning of the *non-maleficence* principle comes into dispute. It may be that a doctor would like to prescribe pethidine for analgesia in labour or morphine for a fracture, but effects of the drug include drowsiness and impaired concentration. If the doctor regards pain as the worst harm, and considers it basic good practice to eliminate it whenever possible, whilst his patient cannot bear to lose her intellectual grip, then there can be a major difficulty of care. The doctor who wishes to be 'non-maleficent' has a dilemma. On his terms he will (by omission) cause harm by not treating the patient while on her terms harm will be caused by the treatment itself. There are equivalent difficulties with *beneficence* and *respect for autonomy*.

The existence of such dilemmas has prompted a proliferation of literature in medical ethics attempting ingenious and sophisticated theoretical solutions.[4] Some writers consider autonomy to be the most important principle – the basic principle which should hold sway when several principles conflict – however there is no consensus. Good analysis of human problems in medicine has less to do with appeal to 'moral principles' than to the systematic use of logic and reason to address the multitude of factors which are bound to be relevant.

Against fallacy 4: Ethics is not 'just a matter of opinion'

The fourth fallacy is actually two fallacies combined. These are:

> 1. That ethics is a subjective activity with no objective means of assessment;
>
> 2. That medicine is an objective activity where subjective judgement ultimately has no legitimate role.

It is unlikely that any reader will have felt entirely neutral about the dilemmas of Doctors X and Y. Indeed, it is probable that many will have responded quickly *against* some possible solutions, and that several will have come down

---

4. *Journal of Medical Ethics*. London: IME Publications: *passim*.

firmly in favour of one way forward. However, despite the facts that there are no uncontroversial ethical standards and that people can be convinced of the merits of utterly conflicting answers to dilemmas, it does not follow that ethics is simply a matter of opinion. If this were to be all that there is to ethical analysis there would be little point in a book of this sort – or indeed in any books on ethics. Fortunately, 'gut reactions' are not the whole story – only the start.

Often there are several reasonable answers to a problem, but it is rarely the case that each solution is of exactly equal merit. For instance, there is an obvious difference in quality between the following two solutions to Doctor X's dilemma:

(a) Doctor X should negotiate calmly and rationally with the male patient in order to encourage him to inform his wife.
(b) Doctor X should immediately threaten that if the man does not tell his wife then he will make the infection public knowledge within the hour.

Usually it can be shown how various proposed solutions can be ranked in some order from best to worst, and the way to show this ranking is not an appeal to intuition, prejudice or rhetoric, but to sustained, credible argument, and to facts both actual and probable. The doctor's job is to learn how to reach and to justify (i.e. to demonstrate to herself and so to others) the best possible solution to a problem in the prevailing circumstances. In this, ethical deliberation can be seen to have a great deal in common with the process of clinical decision making itself. In medicine it is a rare case where there is only one possible diagnosis, a single treatment option, and an entirely uncontroversial programme of management. 'Clinical decisions' are made by taking into account a range of factors: factual, technical, and human. Whether a doctor approaches a case from a 'clinical' or an 'ethical' perspective he must, for a large part of the deliberation, use a similar reasoning process.

Every example in this casebook demonstrates this fact. If ethics is just a matter of opinion then so is medicine. The challenge for doctors who wish to apply ethical analysis to their daily work is to unite two substantial traditions which are often, at present, artificially separated. Just as clinical decision making draws upon a rich history of research, case studies and critical analysis, so does ethical analysis. Neither disciplines have access to absolute certainty but both have well-held principles and conventions of practice on which to draw. The principles of either discipline may be overturned, at least temporarily, in the light of new evidence or ideas.

A More Accurate Picture of Ethics in Medicine

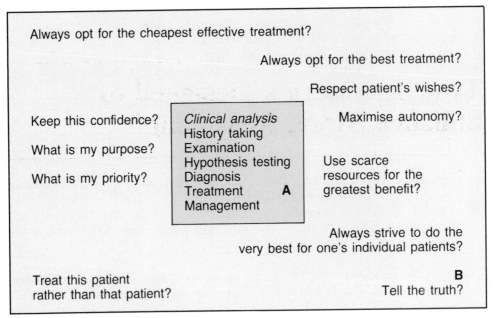

Fig. 2 Ethics in medicine – an essential analytical base; boxes A and B are *inter*dependent

Although pictured here in a very rudimentary way it is more accurate to think of ethics in medicine like this. If human aspects are considered to be at all important, analysis carried out within Box A must always be informed by many other considerations (a few of which are listed in Box B). Since medicine seeks to help unique individuals in complex social environments it is self-evident that the 'clinical process' must be set in a broader base.

This book argues that *ethics* ought to be recognised as that base (the entire content of the Ethical Grid might be transferred to Box B). Through the discussion of real life examples the book demonstrates the fact that skill in ethical analysis is a prerequisite for the best health care.

Two Instruments Designed to Enhance Moral Reasoning⋆

⋆The expressions 'moral reasoning' and 'ethical analysis' can be used interchangeably.

The Ethical Grid

Basic Introduction

The Ethical Grid is a device made up of boxes divided into four layers of different colours. It can help remind the clinician of the range of considerations which might affect his deliberation. In addition it can simplify the process of ethical analysis and help the doctor justify the eventual decision.

The Grid is a distillation of a number of theories of morality and health. As such it should be thought of as a precis of the elements necessary for thorough moral reasoning in health care situations. The Grid assumes that *all* interventions in human health care have definite moral content.

The aim

In using the Grid the doctor's aim must be to select the box or boxes which best solve the problem in hand.

The process

Although it will rarely be necessary to consider a problem of intervention making use of every box, *it is important to consider each situation in the light of each coloured layer.* In other words, before suggesting a solution to a clinical problem affecting one or more people it is crucial for the doctor to take account of:

1. The *principles behind health work* (blue);

2. The *duties* he believes he has (red);

3. The general nature of the *outcome* to be achieved (green);

4. The pertinent *practical features* (black).

In one sense the Grid is merely a reminder that there are at least four separate levels at which to think, and that within these levels there are several different ways of deciding on strategy. As the Grid is used it soon becomes apparent that it is not the Grid that is working – but the doctor. To say 'I am using the Ethical Grid' is simply to say 'I am engaged in moral reasoning'.

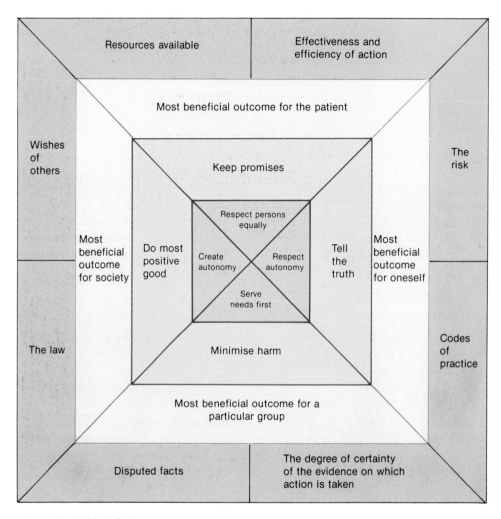

Fig. 3 The Ethical Grid

Each box of the Grid should be thought of as detachable, as if made up of separate plastic chips or wooden blocks.

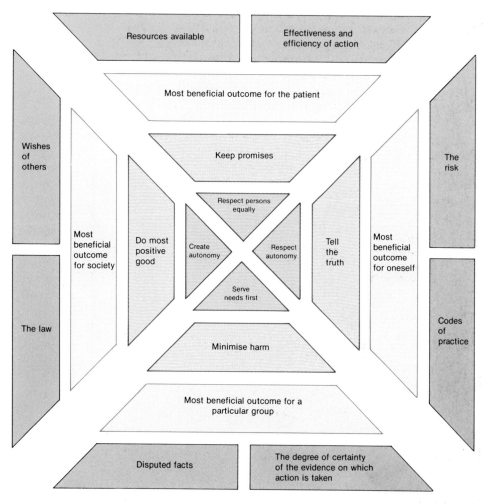

Fig. 4 Each box is detachable

In choosing some boxes, and discarding others, the user will have undertaken a decision-making process and will be able to refer to the boxes selected as 'a record', to enable him to justify his solution to himself, or to other people.

For instance, if a surgeon is faced with a decision about whether or not to perform an operation on an informed patient where the risks and benefits seem to hang in the balance he might, after an extensive period of deliberation, select these boxes:

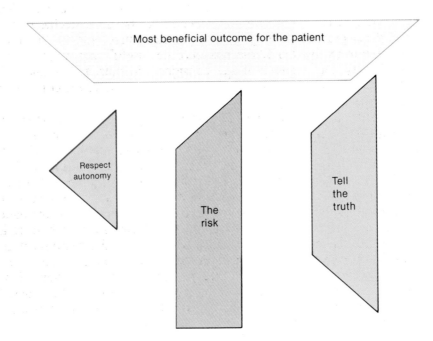

Fig. 5 A selection of boxes after deliberation

These boxes would then act as a reminder of his primary considerations, and of his reasoning and justification of them. The four boxes remind this doctor that he decided to explain every possibility to the patient (**tell the truth**), despite the fact that this could cause anxiety; to abide by the patient's choice (**respect autonomy**); to concentrate only on the needs and desires of the particular patient (**most beneficial outcome for the patient**) and not to consider other patients in the calculation, nor to involve the patient's family; and to try to reduce all material dangers as far as possible (**the risk**).

The Content of the Grid

Black: The level of practicality

Medicine is essentially a practical discipline, and as such it will be a very unusual problem which can be debated without reference to pragmatics. These considerations are represented by the black layer. This layer of the Grid draws attention to **resources available, effectiveness and efficiency of action, the**

risk, **codes of practice, the degree of certainty of the evidence on which
action is taken, disputed facts, the law,** and **wishes of others**.

The words and phrases contained within the boxes in the black level are
essentially nothing more than symbols on paper, as is the case with every box
of the Grid. They require interpretation in order to spring to life, and the
interpretations they are given will vary dependent upon the reasoner and on
the particular context. So, for instance, if it is the task of a General Practitioner
to reach the best possible outcome in a case where he must decide between
computerising his practice or employing a practice nurse, and he 'homes in'
on the box **resources available**, the box becomes useful only when he gives
it meaning. The type of resource under consideration must be specified. For
example, the doctor must be clear whether the resource in question is finance,
talent, personnel or time.

To take an alternative illustration, Doctor Q has already told a patient and
his relatives a certain amount about his condition, but not everything. She is
wondering how best to proceed, and decides to consider the box labelled **the
law**. Dependent on the actual circumstances Doctor Q's attention might be
drawn to different aspects of the law. For instance, it is possible that she may
have revealed more about the patient's condition to the relatives than to the
patient himself. And, on realising that it has become inevitable that the patient
will discover the well-intentioned deception, the doctor may wish to reflect
upon the law as it relates to *breach of confidentiality*.[5] Alternatively, it may
remain possible for the doctor to maintain her 'white lie', but only if in so
doing she keeps some of the risks of therapy secret from the patient. If this
is the case then the doctor, whilst remaining in the box **the law**, may be
interested in a different branch of law – probably the law which relates to
consent and the *tort of negligence* (see Cases 7 and 8).

Green: The level of consequences

Four boxes make up the green layer of the Ethical Grid – the level which is
explicitly concerned with consequences. They are **most beneficial outcome
for the patient, most beneficial outcome for oneself, most beneficial outcome
for society,** and **most beneficial outcome for a particular group**.

The point of including the green layer is to draw attention to the fact that,
whatever decision is taken, although it is likely to produce consequences for
several people or groups of people, one particular set will usually be at the
forefront of any justification. Thus if a doctor decides that he must make it
public knowledge that a patient has been found on testing to be HIV-positive
– even though the patient does not agree to disclosure – then that doctor has
chosen to place what he perceives to be the **most beneficial outcome for
society** before the **most beneficial outcome for the patient** (as perceived by
the patient). The green layer helps clarify what type of outcome is the desired
priority. However, in any case where doctor and patient disagree – or indeed

---

5. Kennedy, I. and Grubb, A. (1989) *Medical Law: Texts and Materials*. London: Butterworths.

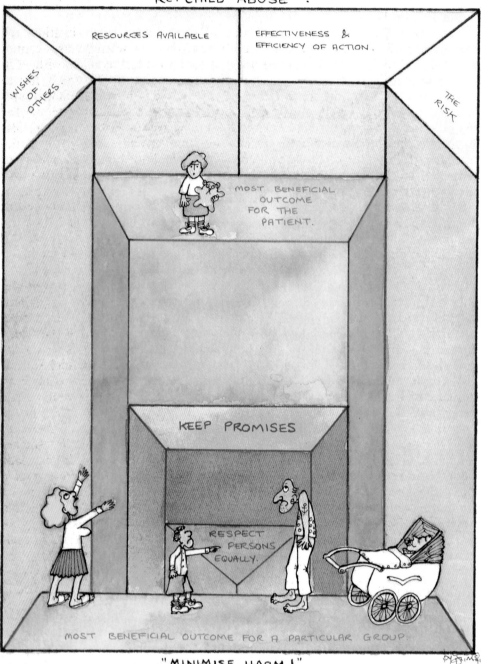

where there is any doubt at all – boxes from other layers must inevitably enter the deliberation.

The above case provides illustration of the point that in some situations the various boxes throughout the Grid – both within and between layers – cannot be used together since they sometimes come into direct conflict with each other. This is quite common. To give a further example, Doctor Z has to deliberate over the human costs and benefits in a case of suspected child abuse, and finds herself unable to select both the box **most beneficial outcome for the patient** and the box **most beneficial outcome for a particular group**. She interprets **the patient** to be the child, and **the particular group** to be the family, and does not think that she can select out both boxes. It appears to Doctor Z that it is probable that to remove the child to a place of safety will cause the family to disintegrate (and that this is undesirable). Of course, it may turn out that the break up of the family actually benefits all concerned, in which case both boxes might have been selected without conflict.

Red: The level of duties

The red layer acts to highlight the notion of 'professional duty'. It is possible, on reading the literature on medical ethics, to discover a host of duties that various authors believe to be incumbent upon doctors. The red layer emphasises only those which are most common. These are **keep promises, tell the truth, minimise harm**, and **do most positive good**. None of these duties should be thought of as binding but all ought at least to be candidates for inclusion in the justification of any decision. However, red boxes, just like black and green boxes, can be excluded from the final selection if this is acceptable to the moral analyst.

Whilst the duties of **promise-keeping** and **truth-telling** need no elaboration at this point, **minimise harm** and **do most positive good** require further explanation. As they stand both expressions are very general but can be made more concrete by thinking of the former as **safety first** – as indicative of a policy where any risks should be minimised as a priority – and the latter as a counterpoise to this strategy. So, in contrast, to **minimise harm**, the dictum **do most positive good** might be thought of as a potential obligation to take risks if there is a chance that by so doing people will be more enabled in their lives.

Blue: The basis of health care

The boxes coloured in blue are the most important in the Ethical Grid. They indicate reasons which are held by some to be the basic inspiration of health care. They are **create autonomy, respect persons equally, respect autonomy**, and **serve needs first**. The blue boxes stand on the following basic justification.

Think of any clinical practice done by a doctor to a patient. Although there might be some disagreement about the best way to carry out the intervention (as the cases discussed in this book show), to a significant extent the action of the doctor will always be inspired by the wish to enable the patient to live in a less impeded state. If not then the doctor's practice will be highly questionable. In other words, a fundamental inspiration of medical care can be seen to be the will to **create autonomy**, the desire to give a person heightened control over his life. Treating a bacterial infection, setting a broken wrist, and counselling an emotionally disturbed man are all standard medical interventions. They are so commonplace that it is hardly ever thought worth asking *why* they are done. But when the question is asked and considered it becomes apparent that the interactions are done for *two* primary motives. On a practical level the interventions are made to relieve discomfort and to restore individuals to states where they are free of disease, injury or illness. But at a deeper level they are made to assist the *development* of human beings in various respects. True health care interventions are made to remove obstacles to various human potentials – physical, intellectual, and emotional – to **create autonomy**.

Since the motivation to **create autonomy** is a fundamental element of medical practice it follows that in areas of their lives where people have adequate autonomy – for instance, in their capacity to make decisions – then that autonomy ought to be respected by doctors. It is often argued that if a person understands the implications of what he wishes to do or to have done to him then a doctor should **respect his autonomous choice** even if he does not agree with it. Once again, as several of the case studies show, medical practice can create difficult conflicts of autonomy (used in the sense of 'ability to choose') – where the choices of the doctor and the patient clash, or where the choices of different patients are in competition. But, as a guide, it is important to remember that unless there are good reasons not to, all decision making with patients should begin from their wishes. It may be that the patient asks the doctor to take charge, to assume full responsibility for decision making. In this case the doctor who takes the blue boxes seriously will agree to act as an 'agent' for the patient, but only if he is satisfied that the maximum possible degree of **autonomy** has first been **created** in the patient.

The blue box **respect persons equally** asserts a traditional assumption of medical practice that, whenever possible – and particularly where the clinical considerations are roughly equivalent – patients should be treated equally, without discrimination. Since all patients share in the human condition, decisions to help one person and not another cannot be taken lightly and must be made – if at all – only after comprehensive deliberation. Consequently an analysis which chooses to exclude this box (as with any of the blue boxes) will require a substantial justification by the moral reasoner. In a similar way the box **serve needs first** is a reminder that when priorities have to be decided in medicine then it is the most needy patients who should be helped first. Thus, if a surgeon has time to treat only one of two patients and one requires life-saving surgery whilst the other has requested only a minor operation, then the former ought to be operated on first. Once again, in practice it is hardly ever as simple as this (see Case 10), but as a basic guide, as a starting point for deliberation, **serve needs first** is a valuable dictum. And if one patient's minor cosmetic surgery comes to take precedence over another patient's hip replacement operation then it can be argued that priorities in medicine have become seriously distorted.

It is important to emphasise that the blue boxes contain various assumptions which cannot be properly justified here (see references 6, 7, 8 and 9 for more detail). In fact they stem from detailed and extensive philosophical research. However, since the Grid is a flexible device which is meant to be fairly freely interpreted by the user, it is possible to invoke these boxes without necessarily accepting the philosophy from which they originated.

Using the Ethical Grid

There are various possible ways of using the Grid. The manner of use preferred depends ultimately on the person who is to use it. However, the following use is recommended:

1. Consider the problem without reference to the Grid. Try to appreciate the extent of the ramifications of possible action. Clarify the issue by listing its key aspects. Attempt to list basic pros and cons of the various options for action.

2. Arrive at an intuitive initial position to a *specifically expressed question.*

3. Consider the Grid in order to test the strength of your position. Consider first the layer felt to be the most significant. This will often be the blue layer since this layer contains the rationale of work for health, and **no genuine health work intervention can ignore every box of the blue layer.** However, users of the Grid will, with experience, develop their own preferences and methodology.

4. Consider all other levels of the Grid, selecting – after appropriate weighing and balancing – those boxes which seem most likely to produce the best possible outcome (create the **highest degree of morality).**

5. Arrange the boxes 'over' the problem to be solved. That is, apply them to your mental picture of the proposed intervention. In this way a course of action will have been decided, and the means to justify it in moral terms will be available.

6. Seedhouse, D.F. (1986) *Health: The Foundations for Achievement.* Chichester: John Wiley and Sons.
7. Seedhouse, D.F. (1988) *Ethics: The Heart of Health Care.* Chichester: John Wiley and Sons.
8. Seedhouse, D.F. and Cribb, A. (eds) (1989) *Changing Ideas in Health Care.* Chichester: John Wiley and Sons.
9. Seedhouse, D.F. (1991) *Liberating Medicine.* Chichester: John Wiley and Sons.

The limit to the use of the Grid

It might seem that the Grid is so flexible that it can be used to justify any solution to any dilemma. But this is not the case. Certain solutions, for instance those which involve unnecessary deception, or manipulation of people, or avoidable pain, cannot be described as *enabling* or *enhancing* and so cannot be justified by recourse to the boxes of the Grid. In addition, not all enabling solutions can be said to be of equal merit. The onus is on the user of the Grid to show how the chosen course of action is to be preferred over any other.

The Grid can be used legitimately only by those who honestly seek to enable life-enhancing human potentials. Consequently the Grid can be used only with integrity. If it is used insincerely, if the Grid is employed cynically – merely to get results in order to further some selfish goal, for instance, then this is not a moral use, even though the outcomes might not be significantly different from those resulting from sincere use.

The Algorithm

The Algorithm has been derived from the Grid. It must be used in a more systematic way than its parent. However, although it is less flexible, its step by step approach ensures that the moral reasoning process is always thorough. Some doctors will find the Algorithm restrictive in its insistence on procedure, but others will welcome the guidance, particularly whilst novices in the skill of moral reasoning.

The Algorithm is divided into four quadrants which are equivalent to the four coloured layers of the Grid. The user must begin in the quadrant which seems to hold most immediate relevance to her. The Algorithm allows the user to circle until she decides to leave and move to the **Final Common Pathway**. This limited flexibility allows her to reconsider any quadrant in the light of new information or conclusions which have arisen during analysis of the other quadrants. Once on the **Final Common Pathway** the user still has the option of returning to the Algorithm. If she does not, then she must make her final decision about the problem.

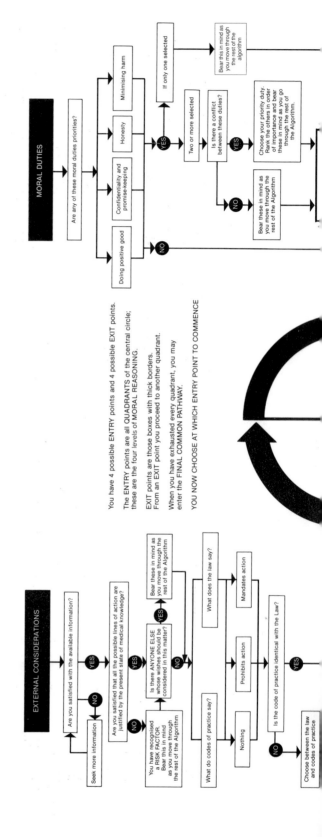

You have 4 possible ENTRY points and 4 possible EXIT points.

The ENTRY points are all QUADRANTS of the central circle; these are the four levels of MORAL REASONING.

EXIT points are those boxes with thick borders. From an EXIT point you proceed to another quadrant.

When you have exhausted every quadrant, you may enter the FINAL COMMON PATHWAY.

YOU NOW CHOOSE AT WHICH ENTRY POINT TO COMMENCE

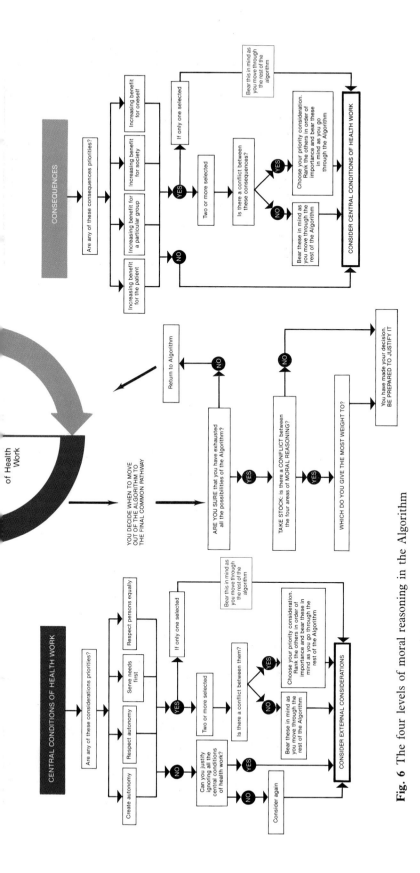

Fig. 6 The four levels of moral reasoning in the Algorithm

The Cases

How to Use this Casebook

The 15 cases described in this book have been arranged so as to illustrate the use of the decision-making tools in the most accessible way. Potentially each situation is enormously complicated, but all have been kept within realistic bounds. The earliest cases are described in the simplest possible way in order to show how the Grid and Algorithm might be used to produce a practical result. Most of the later cases are more discursive, and are presented in a manner designed to open up productive thinking and group discussion. If this casebook is to be used for a series of classes it is recommended that the cases are considered in the order they are presented below. Once the cases have been explored, and the Grid and Algorithm are familiar, doctors should experiment with structured ethical analysis of real cases.

Although it is not expected that on confronting an urgent ethical problem a doctor will instantly refer to this casebook and attempt to apply one of the tools directly, it is hoped that the book will be carried by clinicians for reference whenever time or the nature of a particular case permits.

Case 1

A Dilemma in Casualty

Introduction

Doctors on casualty duty are regularly called upon to make quick decisions where the stakes are high. Whilst it is quite impractical for a doctor to undertake a calm and detailed ethical analysis during a crisis, it can be of great benefit to have thought through the fundamental issues in advance. This case describes one such urgent situation, and relates the thinking of the people involved to some of the categories of the Ethical Grid.

The situation

A middle-aged man, Derek Coles, has been brought into a Casualty Department by the police, who have found him lying on a pavement in a residential area. He is very distressed and tells staff that he has taken a large bottle of paracetamol steadily over the last few hours. He refuses all offers of treatment.

Arguments for and against treating the man against his will are outlined below.

Stage One: Response to Crisis

In favour of treatment

Dr O'Brien, the casualty officer on duty, has come across a similar situation before and is clear about her position. Using the Ethical Grid as her point of reference, she believes that the answer must depend on adherence to the principles laid out in the red level, since she sees the solution to be based in *duty*.

Derek Coles is not very large and by now somewhat drowsy. She knows that if no treatment is offered then the **consequences** (green) will almost certainly be death. Dr O'Brien is unable to understand how Mr Coles' death will **increase benefit** (green) for anybody, including himself. She knows too that she is not psychologically equipped simply to stand back and watch a human being die. Dr O'Brien is of the firm opinion that health workers have a basic obligation both to **do positive good** (red) and to **minimise harm** (red) on every occasion and in any circumstance. It is clear to her that these general goals can be achieved in this particular case only through treating Mr Coles.

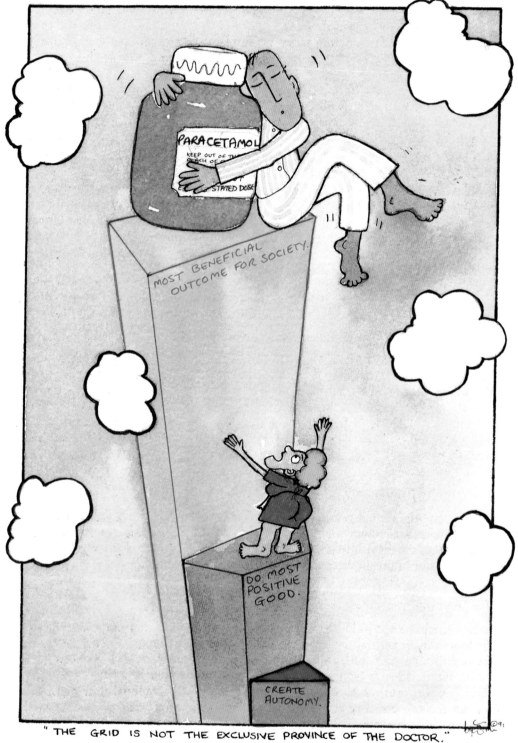

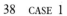

A stomach washout and an emetic will almost certainly clear most of the paracetamol from the patient's stomach. If necessary repeated doses of methionine could be forced down.

Under common law, doctors have the right to treat in an emergency if they believe that by doing so they are acting in the best interests of the patient. However, the doctor is by no means entirely free to act on her beliefs. It is illegal for doctors even to touch a person without that person's consent. To do so would be to risk an action in battery. Derek has not attended voluntarily, and does not want to be treated. Theoretically he is at liberty to leave. Dr O'Brien's best hope of success is that the patient becomes unconscious in the Department, before it is too late to give the antidote. She might then treat him as an emergency case, although her security in law would be far from certain since the patient has consistently refused consent whilst conscious (see below).

Against treatment

Derek feels he has good cause to be depressed. He has lost his job, is £2000 in debt, and in trouble with money lenders. He can see no escape from this predicament other than to take his own life. He is afraid that the creditors will harm his family if he does not pay them. At least if he is dead there is less chance that his family will suffer for his inadequacies. If Derek were to be in a position to argue with help from the Grid (which is not the exclusive province of doctors) it is likely that he would focus on the green and blue levels. He is convinced that the consequences of his death will be the **most beneficial outcome** (green) for him (a release from so much that is negative can only be good), and so also for his family. He is asserting his basic right to decide what to do with his life. Throughout his 'detention' he has been quite consistent that everyone, doctors included, should **respect his wishes** (blue).

Stage Two: What Next?

The situation has developed. Despite the ethical and legal uncertainty, Dr O'Brien has done all she can to detoxify her patient. She is now faced with the problem of his further management. She calls the psychiatrist on duty and asks for his opinion of the patient, with a view to admission.

The psychiatrist's response

As he recovers physically Derek explains his predicament to the psychiatrist, who assesses his mental state. The doctor is familiar with the Ethical Grid and knows he must *formulate and address a clear question* to use it properly (see p. 27). He decides to ask: *should I allow this man to leave hospital or should I detain him for further assessment?* He thinks first about potential outcomes. He ponders the consequences of letting Derek leave hospital in his present mental state, and quickly concludes that Derek would be at high risk of a further suicide attempt. He does not agree with Derek that his death would be in his best interests or those of his family, and tells him so. Neither can the psychiatrist see any **benefit** (green) resulting from an immediate discharge.

Up to this point the psychiatrist has not queried Derek's story. Can he be sure of the patient's account? In other words, what is **the degree of certainty of the evidence on which action is to be taken** (black)? The psychiatrist already suspects that Derek may have a depressive disorder and he knows that *ideas of poverty* and *paranoid ideas* can present as symptoms of the condition. If Derek does have a mental disorder this could impair his ability to make rational decisions. The psychiatrist is of the opinion that it is less than rational to think of suicide as a panacea for Derek's real or imaginary family problems. He decides to use this interpretation of Derek's actions to justify ignoring the blue box **respect autonomy**, since he believes that Derek's disorder seriously undermines his ability to choose sensibly. However, the consultant does not disregard the entire blue level since he believes that Derek has a **need** of life, not death, and that he can be cured. And, he believes, curing people to **create** more **autonomy** (blue) is the whole purpose of medicine.

The psychiatrist admits inwardly that he is not certain at this stage whether Derek does indeed have a mental disorder or, if he does, whether this is impairing his rationality. However, focusing again on the black layer, he feels that the overall **risk** (black) of letting Derek leave immediately is too high. He decides he needs more time to assess Derek than the hour he has spent with him in casualty. Thus he feels justified in recommending his detention for further assessment under Section 2 of the Mental Health Act 1983.

During his analysis the consultant psychiatrist selected from the Grid the boxes **most beneficial outcome for a particular group** (which he defined as Derek's family), **most beneficial outcome for the patient, the degree of certainty of the evidence on which action is taken, the risk** and **create autonomy**. In this way he has reasoned systematically, he has covered a number of key aspects, he has listed the basic components of his decision, and he has a record to help him justify his ethical analysis to others if necessary.

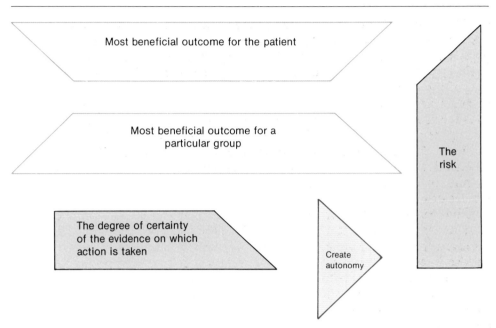

Fig. 7 The boxes selected by the psychiatrist

EXERCISE

It may be that you disagree with the doctors' justifications. If so, state and attempt to justify, using the Grid, an alternative way of dealing with the situation.

If you do agree with the two medical assessments then attempt a different exercise. Instead, try to use the Grid to justify a policy that in every imaginable case a doctor ought to treat a person to prevent a suicide. Before you do so read carefully the legal notes which you will find below.

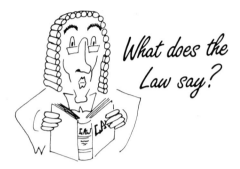

What does the Law say?

Hoggett in *Mental Health Law* (1984), pp 201–203, writes:

As suicide is no longer a crime, can he be prevented from carrying out his intention even if he is not 'insane' within the meaning of the common law power to restrain? And if he has succeeded in poisoning or otherwise attacking himself, can steps be taken to save his life against his will and without sectioning him?

Taken to its logical conclusion, such a doctrine would allow us to overrule the protests of any patient, sane or insane, who wished to decline such treatment (for example, the Jehovah's Witness who had conscientious objections to a life-saving blood transfusion; or the elderly person who no longer wished for massive surgical attempts to prolong life).

The most we can be absolutely sure of is this. The doctor may proceed where the treatment is 'necessary', in the sense that the patient may die or suffer serious harm if it is postponed until he can be consulted, but only where it is reasonable to assume that the patient would have consented, in other words where he is not known to object. We may also be tolerably certain that the law would not condemn intervention which is absolutely necessary to save the patient's life in some cases where he is known to object. This must be true of the attempted suicide, where in any event it is possible to argue that he did not genuinely wish to succeed, but it is far less obviously true of the known Jehovah's Witness who requires a blood transfusion. In all these cases, however, even if there is a technical battery, no jury is likely to convict, and there could be no substantial damages for 'wrongful life'.

But we cannot be sure how much further these principles will carry us, particularly in relation to patients who are permanently incapable of giving or withholding their consent.

[The example of Professor Hoggett's based upon a Jehovah's Witness who is given a blood transfusion whilst unconscious arose in the Ontario case of *Malette v Shulman* (21 December 1987, unreported) where the defendant ignored a clear written instruction not to transfuse the plaintiff. The plaintiff successfully sued the doctor in battery and recovered $20,000 (Canadian).]

continued

continued

Skegg in *Law, Ethics and Medicine* (1984), pp 110–113, writes:

In all but the most exceptional circumstances, a doctor may not carry out treatment involving the bodily touching of a patient who is capable of consenting, if the patient's consent has not been sought, or if the patient has refused to give consent. The fact that, without the treatment, the patient's health will suffer will not of itself justify a doctor in overriding the patient's refusal. Indeed, in many circumstances, even the certainty that the patient will die if treatment is not given will not justify a doctor in proceeding without consent.

However, there is at least one exception to the general rule that consent is required. Where someone has done something in an apparent attempt to kill himself, doctors will often be justified in taking action to avert the consequences of that action. Prior to the abolition of the offence of suicide, there was no difficulty in explaining the legal basis for a doctor acting to prevent a person from attempting to commit suicide, or to avoid death resulting from such an attempt. Suicide was a felony, so the doctor was simply exercising the general liberty to prevent a felony. Doctors were not only free to prevent someone from committing suicide; they were sometimes under a duty to do so. However, since the enactment of the Suicide Act 1961 it has continued to be accepted that doctors are sometimes free – sometimes, indeed, under a duty – to prevent patients from committing suicide.

In some cases, the person who has apparently attempted to commit suicide will be suffering from a mental disorder which prevents the giving or withholding of consent. But in many cases the person will have a sufficient understanding to give, or withhold, consent. This is so, even though the act will often result from a passing impulse or temporary depression, rather than from a rational and fixed decision. If restrained and given assistance, the majority are glad that their action did not result in death. Hence, even if it is accepted that a person should not be prevented from carrying out a calm or a reasoned decision to terminate his own life, there is an overwhelming case for intervention where there is reason to believe that, if given help, the person will be glad he did not kill, or seriously injure, himself. Doctors are constantly intervening in these circumstances and there can be little doubt that, were their conduct to be questioned, the courts would hold it justified.

Kennedy, I. and Grubb, A. (1989) *Medical Law: Texts and Materials*, pp 293–4 and 348. London: Butterworths.

Case 2

Should I '. . . Respect the Secrets which Are Confided in Me . . .'?

Introduction

Coming early in the casebook this case is relatively sparsely analysed. It is written in the second person singular. 'You' are taken through the case as if you were making use of the Algorithm. Of course, it may be that you would not choose to reason in this way, in which case you should analyse the situation with the Algorithm and substitute your own judgements for those described below.

The situation

You are a genetic counsellor. It has been discovered that one of your patients is affected by an autosomal dominant condition of variable penetrance (tuberous sclerosis*). You request permission to inform the patient's sister via her doctor since there is a high chance that she too will be affected. Your patient refuses.

What do you do in such circumstances? How might you use the Algorithm to assist your thinking?

Using the Algorithm

You focus first on the quadrant Moral Duties (red) and decide that **confidentiality and promise-keeping**, and **minimising harm** are important duties to consider in this situation. In order to **minimise harm** you feel that you ought to tell your patient's sister about the risk of her bearing an affected child. Of course you are aware that if you do this you will break your **promise of confidentiality** to your patient. You see that there is a conflict between these duties. On reflection you decide that the duty to maintain **confidentiality**

---

*This genetically determined condition is inherited as an autosomal dominant, but is variable in its expression among individuals carrying the disorder. Families have been described, for example, where a mother has some of the stigmata (a diagnostic butterfly rash on the face), but is herself neither disabled nor handicapped. She, however, has children who are both disabled and handicapped (often to very different degrees). The extent to which the gene for this condition expresses itself appears to be extremely variable. Having the disorder, being disabled by it and being mentally handicapped are three quite separate and distinct situations.[1]

ought to take priority because it was made directly to a patient, whereas you feel that you have less responsibility towards the sister. This is a tentative decision which you are quite prepared to overturn as you travel through the Algorithm.

You make a note of your provisional position and move on to consider the Consequences (green) of abiding by your patient's wishes. On studying the available boxes you select three as initial priorities: **increasing benefit for the patient, increasing benefit for a particular group**, and **increasing benefit for society**.

Just as is the case with the Grid, each of these boxes requires interpretation. It is essential that you specify what is to count as 'benefit' in the situation. If, for example, you choose to take benefit to mean *enabling people to carry out chosen courses of action* then this will have different implications than if benefit were taken to mean *decreasing the chances of handicapped children being born*. In a case such as this, where several boxes are potentially important, and where different interpretations of 'benefit' seem potentially relevant, you must think deeply, and will certainly need to continue to circle within the Algorithm in order to clarify your thinking about desirable outcomes.

In this analysis you eventually decide that the central consequence which you must take into account is **damage**. Thus benefit might be increased in so far as **damage** is prevented or minimised. You have already decided not to **damage** your relationship with the patient by breaking a confidence (and so also not to damage the trust of future clients), but now you wonder – thinking more directly about outcome rather than duty – whether or not a life lived suffering from handicap, and a mother burdened with coping with such a life, is not a more central **damage** in this case. In addition, you reflect, a handicapped child imposes a significant financial burden on society – to prevent the birth of a damaged child could be to **increase benefit for society**.

At the stage you have reached you are faced with a conflict between your perceived duty of confidence to the patient, and your concern to prevent the various other **damages** happening. This problem must be resolved, so you turn to the quadrant Central Conditions of Health Work (blue). You are clear that you wish to **respect your patient's autonomy**. But in doing this you cannot **respect persons equally** because you would be giving preferential care to the patient above her sister. Of course, if you override the wishes of your patient you will exhibit bias in the other direction. Whatever decision you make you will have to offend against the principle **respect persons equally**. It seems that you cannot win. Moreover, by **respecting your patient's autonomy** you are in effect impeding rather than **creating** the **autonomy** of her sibling. Is it more important to **respect your patient's autonomy** than **create autonomy** for her sister? Tentatively, you decide that it is.

On scanning the notes you have made so far you see that you have oscillated in your thinking as you have progressed through the Algorithm. First you felt that you had a duty (red) to keep a promise to your patient, then you believed that the potential bad consequences (green) overrode this duty, and now you have moved back to your original position. Not to respect the reasoned choice of a person for whom you are meant to care would be a decision of considerable import – one not to be taken lightly. But you are still far from sure.

You review the External Considerations (black). You are quite satisfied with the **evidence** suggesting that your patient has tuberous sclerosis but why does she not want her sister to know? Malice? Protectiveness? Guilt? Shame? Embarrassment? You press on with your counselling and discover that the sister is about to marry, and is 16 weeks pregnant. Your patient is convinced that if her sister learns about this condition she will be bound to tell her fiancé, who will then break off the engagement. This may or may not be true, but you now have a more realistic picture of the potential ramifications of any decision that you or the patient might make. Certainly there are **other** people involved whose **wishes** ought to be taken into account – the trouble is that you don't know what these wishes are. In addition, although you know that your patient has tuberous sclerosis you cannot be sure to what extent her sister's child would be affected. Such a child could have anything from severe mental handicap to mild stigmata of the disease.

You consider the BMA's **code of practice** on genetic counselling. This argues that your patient's sister, because she is almost certainly affected – although probably by a mild form of the disease – is entitled to the information despite your patient's wishes. Does **the law** add anything? The Court of Appeal has held that information obtained in a confidential relationship may be disclosed if in the public interest. It seems to you at least a possibility that the potential prevention of the birth of a damaged child could be considered sufficient to merit disclosure. It looks as if both **the law** and your **code of practice** would support you should you decide to ignore your patient's wishes.

You review each quadrant again. You still think that there is a pressing duty of **confidentiality**, and you have regard for the principle of **respect for autonomy**. Against this you weigh up the consequences for others of abiding by this duty. You have already acknowledged that the patient's sister may suffer distress, and now you know that there is an unborn child and fiancé to consider. It is not too late for the sister to have an abortion if that is her wish. What is more she might even have a case in negligence against you for failing in your duty to warn her of a foreseeable risk.[2]

You take stock: **confidentiality** and **respect for patient autonomy** against the **consequences** to the patient's sister, her fiancé and society. On balance you decide that the latter considerations prevail. You feel supported in this decision by the law and your professional body. Consequently, you make sure that the patient's sister is told.

EXERCISE

Consider this problem yourself with the help of the Algorithm. Would you use the Algorithm differently?

References

1. Russell, O. (1985) *Current Reviews in Psychiatry: Mental Handicap.* Churchill-Livingstone.
2. Tarasoff v Regents of the University of California, 529 P2d 553, 118 Cal Rptr 129 (Cal Sup Ct 1974).

Case 3

Euthanasia

Introduction

Euthanasia is perhaps the oldest issue in medical ethics. We all must die but, given the choice, very few of us would choose to die in pain. Naturally we would rather avoid physical, emotional or social distress if at all possible. But does this fact of human life mean that it is therefore right that death should be hastened?

There are many points of view on this question, and many practical, ethical, and legal factors to be taken into account whenever it is raised. Numerous doctors and philosophers have studied and dissected the topic of euthanasia. This work has produced a number of definitions and classification types.

Definitions and distinctions

Some definitions and distinctions are commonly made in the 'euthanasia debate', although their precise content is often disputed. For example, there is continuing controversy over the distinction between 'active' and 'passive' euthanasia. It is said by some that there is a difference between *active euthanasia* (which means to do something positive, such as administering a lethal dose of barbiturates, to end a life) and *passive euthanasia* (which means to do nothing to save a life when that life might have been saved: for example, not to treat pneumonia with antibiotics, as is suggested in the case described below). Others insist that either there is no difference at all, or only a difference of scale. However, there is a fairly general agreement that *euthanasia* means a 'good/gentle/easy death' or, more precisely, to 'kill someone where, on account of his distressing physical or mental state, this is thought to be in his own interests'.

The standard definition of *voluntary euthanasia* is 'to end a life on the request of the person who wishes to die, when that person is unable to commit suicide'. For example, a person who is psychologically unable to inject herself, or who is paralysed by an illness such as multiple sclerosis, might volunteer for euthanasia. *Non-voluntary euthanasia* means to kill someone, in his own interests, where he is either not in a position to have, or not in a position to express, any views on the matter. For example, the senile, the totally paralysed, and severely handicapped babies might be considered for non-voluntary euthanasia. *Involuntary euthanasia* is the most radical type. Its definition is 'to kill someone, in his own interests, in disregard of his own views'. For example, to kill him without finding out what he thinks, or to kill him against his expressed preference: perhaps a person is in terrible pain, cannot communicate, but has said previously that he would wish to live for as long as possible. When there is no longer any way to establish whether or not his view has changed, and euthanasia is carried out, then this would seem to be a case of involuntary rather than non-voluntary euthanasia. *Assisted suicide* means enabling a person to take the necessary steps to kill herself.

The notion of *double-effect* is often referred to in euthanasia debates. The double-effect argument is used to justify euthanasia by distinguishing between the supposed primary and secondary effects of treatment – between intended and unintended (but foreseeable) consequences. So, it is argued, if the primary intention of medical activity is to relieve a person's pain, which necessitates a dangerously high dosage of morphine, and this has the 'secondary effect' of causing death (not intended), then this is morally justified. This notion can be of great psychological help to a carer who has to make this sort of choice, although it is of dubious philosophical validity.

Alternatives

Jonathan Glover[1] has outlined five discrete alternatives for doctors in situations where euthanasia might be an option:

1. To take all possible steps to preserve life.
2. To take all 'ordinary' steps to preserve life, but not to use 'extraordinary' means. (With this option it is necessary to define 'ordinary' and 'extraordinary', and this cannot be done without controversy. A rule of thumb guideline to this distinction is to ask, 'do the likely results justify the drawbacks of the methods?' So, if the therapy under consideration is likely to be expensive, unusual, difficult, painful or dangerous then it might be said to be 'extraordinary'. On this definition the treatment of pneumonia in the case below by antibiotics might arguably be said to be 'ordinary', and its treatment by antibiotics and aggressive physiotherapy 'extraordinary'.)
3. Not to kill, but to take no steps to preserve life.
4. Not to intend to kill but to act in such a way that death might be foreseen as a consequence (double-effect).
5. Deliberately to kill.

This is not the place to discuss such distinctions in detail, although it is helpful to highlight them. Instead, the following case presents a typical real-life problem for a doctor, and suggests routes towards informed and systematic ethical analysis.

The Old Schoolmaster

In August Mr Bill Harley, a 70 year old man, started to notice a marked deterioration in his memory. He found this very frustrating since he had always been proud of his ability to recall facts. In 40 years as a physics teacher he had never once made a mistake over a boy's name.

During the ensuing six months his cognitive faculties worsened considerably – to the point where Bill's doctor advised him never to go out unaccompanied. By this stage he had not been able to find his way back home on three occasions. Dorothy, Bill's wife and three years his senior, was finding him increasingly difficult to care for. She could just about cope with his forgetfulness but his irritability upset her, especially since Bill had always been a kind and tolerant man.

In the end Dorothy managed to care for Bill for two years following the onset of his impairment even though Bill became incontinent, and often failed to recognise her. Then Bill's health deteriorated further. The Harley's GP, Dr Morris, diagnosed pneumonia, upon which he was faced with a painful question: should he treat Bill with appropriate antibiotics, or should he do nothing and 'let nature take its course'?

Dr Morris had been Bill's GP for 30 years and remembered him fondly as an active intelligent man. He also recalled that Bill had told him on a social occasion, although in all seriousness, that should he lose 'his faculties' he would not wish to be a burden on Dorothy and wanted no heroic measures taken to sustain his life. A group of people at a party had been discussing the case of a son of a local businessman who had been injured in a motorbike accident, and was now apparently permanently comatosed. Bill, he remembered, was adamant that a life had to mean something to be worth fighting for. Dr Morris could not quite recall his own position at the time, but guessed that he had sided with Bill.

What should the doctor do? Can the Ethical Grid help?

The doctor's analysis

Dr Morris looks first at the blue layer. He knows that autonomy must be an important issue in this case. But how can he **respect** Bill's **autonomy**? Surely in his present mental state Bill is not an autonomous individual. He cannot participate meaningfully in decision making, especially not in a decision so complicated and important as this. To be sure, Bill indicated in the past that he would not want his life sustained in the type of circumstances he now experiences, but Dr Morris feels he cannot be certain that the Bill who said this some years ago would want to be bound now by that decision. People often change their minds about their desires when confronted with real rather than hypothetical situations. So, reluctantly, he decides to ignore the box **respect autonomy**. Naturally Dr Morris wants to **create autonomy** for any patient in his care but medical science cannot restore Bill's ability to think. Of course, the doctor can prescribe antibiotics, which would stand a fair chance of curing the attack of pneumonia, but would this be to **create autonomy** in any real sense?

Re : EUTHANASIA :

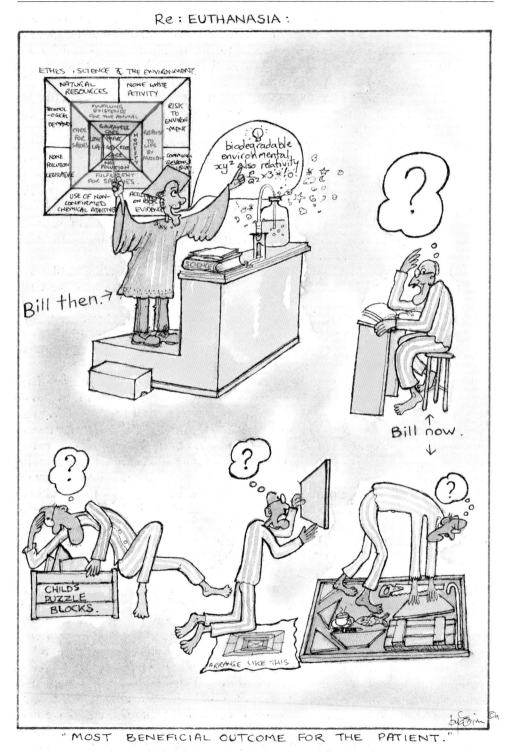

"MOST BENEFICIAL OUTCOME FOR THE PATIENT."

These thoughts lead Dr Morris to consider more closely the consequences of the courses of action open to him. A gentle death might well be in Bill's best interest. Morris reasons that Bill's quality of life is now awful by any standard and is especially hard (for others at least) to bear in a man of such past intelligence and energy. His present state is pitiful and undignified. If the doctor could give him dignity, and peace, then this – rather than suffer the degradation of a dementing illness – might be said to be the **most beneficial outcome for the patient**.

Moreover, Bill's wife has suffered mentally and physically through the effort of caring for him. Dr Morris believes that she would probably be better off without him. And, as always, there is a **resource issue**. If Bill were to die the Practice Nurses could spend more time with other patients. Since the practice assumed its own budget Dr Morris has become increasingly aware of the expense of chronic patients. Furthermore, caring for them seriously saps the morale of his nurses. To let Bill die would be to the economic and general good of his practice, and indirectly to Morris himself.

Dr Morris is becoming convinced that he should not prescribe antibiotics. But does he have any overriding duty? He turns to the red layer of the Grid. He considers that the boxes **minimise harm** and **do most positive good** are relevant to this case. Morris reasons again that he would be harming Bill by prolonging his unhappy existence, and that he would do both Bill and his wife **positive good** by not intervening. He concludes that he would not be contravening his duties as a doctor should he decide not to prescribe.

Finally the doctor turns to the black layer of the Grid, where many of the boxes seem relevant. He has already made a judgement that Dorothy would be better off without her husband but he has not yet checked out her feelings. He does so, sensitively pointing out that Bill could die if left untreated. Dorothy feels abhorrence that a decision she could make might be a partial cause of her husband's death, guilt at her wanting his death, and continuing pain at seeing her husband 'in this state'. She says she 'just doesn't know'. Their son, who has come home from abroad on hearing news of his father's condition, tells Dr Morris that he thinks Bill should not be treated. Dr Morris does not have a consistent directive from Bill's relatives, but believes that Bill's wife, by saying she doesn't know what to do, is indirectly asking him to take on the final responsibility for the decision. He reflects that it is, anyway, perhaps unfair to expect any lay-person to exercise clinical judgement.

Can **the law** or the BMA's **code of practice** carry some of the burden? There is no voluntary euthanasia legislation in the UK – in fact intentionally to take the life of another person is prima facie murder – and the European Convention of Human Rights specifically states that life should not be shortened intentionally. The complexity of the situation is heightened because Bill is incompetent and cannot express a wish. Notable cases in the USA (Karen Quinlan case;[2] Saikewicz case[3]) have addressed the problem of treatment of the mentally incompetent through the court making a 'substituted judgement', that is making a decision for the patient which it is believed would have been made by the patient if he were able. But no such cases exist in British law. Indeed, the Mental Health Act 1983 gives no greater power to doctors to withhold treatment to the mentally incompetent than to other patients.

If Bill were competent then he would have a legal right to refuse any treatment (since consent to treatment is a requirement in law – see Case 1). However, since he is not competent the issue is cloudy – the law does not give Dr Morris a clear and obvious guideline. The BMA[4] is opposed to active voluntary euthanasia, but Dr Morris would not have to act to shorten life. He need only be a passive observer. Given this he thinks that he would probably find his decision not to treat supported by the majority of his professional colleagues.

The doctor's decision

On balance Dr Morris decides not to prescribe in the belief that he is **increasing the good of all** concerned and ought as a doctor to **minimise harm**. He believes that the BMA will support his decision and that he will not be contravening **the law**. Interestingly, he has not selected a box from the blue level (see p. 27 for a comment on such an omission), and neither has he used the Grid in the way suggested in the Introduction.

Possible counter-arguments

Some doctors might argue against Dr Morris along the following lines:

Although Dr Morris may believe Bill's state to be pitiful and undignified, it is paternalistic to assume that Bill's quality of life is so poor that he should be allowed to die, and then to act on this premise. Only Bill can decide whether his life is worth living or not. Doctors must constantly be on the alert not to make a major, albeit understandable, mistake. We all imagine that if we find something enjoyable – or unbearable – that these emotions will be experienced by all other human beings in similar circumstances. But experience shows that this is not so. For instance, some people commit suicide if they lose a person they love, whilst others, apparently in similar pain, choose to continue with their lives. Experience is subjective and is not, ultimately, something which can be assessed objectively. A doctor's task must be to prolong life because this means, at least, that possibilities remain. Even if these possibilities are only to suffer this does not give doctors a right to participate in shortening lives.

Doctors who are more radical still might go further and admit that it is not actually a medical decision at all. Such a group might point out that Dorothy could suffocate Bill with a pillow if she wanted, which could not be described as a medical act. They might add that Dr Morris' decision not to do anything medical is, itself, not a clinical judgement since nothing medical results from it. Of course others might argue that *any* reasoning done by a doctor in his professional role is a clinical judgement, but this is not the place to consider semantic controversy.

EXERCISE

1. Is Dr Morris justified in his decision? Which blue boxes might he have used? Are there any wider implications not considered in the doctor's analysis? Do the counter-arguments carry conviction? How might these arguments be developed?

2. Repeat Dr Morris' original analysis, but this time in exactly the way prescribed in the Introduction. Also, offer the strongest possible justification for not including any blue boxes.

References

1. Glover, J. (1977) *Causing Death and Saving Lives*, p. 195. London: Penguin.
2. In re Quinlan (1976) 355A.2d.647.
3. Superintendent of Belchertown State School v Saikewicz (1977) 370NE. 2d.417.
4. British Medical Association (1981) *The Handbook of Medical Ethics*, p. 35, section 5.28. London: BMA.

Case 4

To Whom Am I Obliged?

Introduction

One of the most common ethical problems for any health worker is to establish which people he has a moral duty to care for, and which for whom he has no professional responsibility. Some doctors argue that the clinician's duty lies only with the patients directly under his charge. Other insist that the obligation of medicine is to serve all people in need regardless of age, gender or race. For these doctors it is morally immaterial whether a person is currently receiving therapy at their hand – what matters is their need.

Both positions pose difficulties. The doctor who feels a duty only towards his own patients must explain what criteria – other than chance – govern his choice. And if it can be shown that there are patients not in his charge who are in more need than those he is treating, then the doctor faces a hard dilemma. Should he cease to help those in relatively less need or must he see their treatment through? The doctor who believes that medicine should be devoted to all people, not just those who happen to be in the closest proximity to him, faces the same dilemma, and is often even less equipped to deal with it. At least the former doctor is able to make a decision based on a promise (made to an individual) to treat until treatment is no longer helpful.

Although the following case does not place the doctor in a position where he must decide who not to *treat* (see Case 15 for a resource allocation problem of this kind), it nevertheless raises the same basic issue: *do I have an obligation to my patient only, or do I have obligations to others not directly in my care? And if I do have obligations to others, do these obligations ever outweigh those I have to my patient?*

Who Comes First?

In this case a doctor finds herself faced with a difficult ethical problem. She asks for assistance from other members of the 'health care team', and receives particular help from two nurse colleagues. Although the study raises striking questions of promise-keeping and truth-telling, it hinges on the question: *what is the extent of the doctor's responsibility?*

The situation

Hilda is 75 years old. She lives with her daughter, Monica, who is a single parent with a nine year old girl. Monica works long hard hours to support her daughter and elderly mother, and has very little time to pursue her own interests or to meet other people.

On several occasions lately Hilda has fallen in the street. Each time she has been helped home by neighbours. Twice she has needed hospital care for injuries sustained in falling. She has also had a series of infections and during a recent bout of 'flu' forgot to light the gas, leaving it on for four hours before a neighbour smelt it and turned it off. Now Hilda has fallen again and been taken to hospital. Following tests it has been found that she has a serious blood condition called acute myeloid leukaemia. She may have only one or two years to live, even with intensive therapy, and there is no cure. Hilda asks Dr Owens, the consultant in charge of her case, to promise that she will tell Monica neither the diagnosis or prognosis because 'she has enough on her plate as it is'. Hilda says that she is not afraid to die and is looking forward to making the most of her last few months at home with her family. Dr Owens agrees to Hilda's request.

Monica visits the hospital under the impression that Hilda's problem is only her fall. But she has reached a personal watershed. This is enough. She says that she really cannot cope with her mother any more – she ought to go into 'a home'. She turns to Dr Owens for help. She asks her to tell Hilda that she is now so frail, from repeated falls, that she will not be able to return home, and that arrangements will have to be made for her to live elsewhere. Dr Owens replies that she appreciates Monica's difficulties but she will have to think about what to do because, strictly speaking, Hilda could be discharged in three days' time.

Dr Owens calls a case conference, worried that she should not have made a promise to Hilda. Two senior nurses offer quite different solutions to Dr Owens. In keeping with hospital policy in case conferences all participants have access to the Ethical Grid.

Nurse Evans

Nurse Evans' general outlook is that health work should enable not only the patients in immediate care but also their families and, as often as possible, the community at large. The essential pattern of her deliberation is outlined below.

As she studied the Grid, Nurse Evans was immediately drawn to the blue layer. She believes that health workers have a fundamental responsibility to **respect autonomy**, but Monica and Hilda seem to have conflicting wishes which cannot be respected simultaneously. Hilda wants to go home; Monica wants Hilda in a home. Hilda wants to keep the truth from Monica, and Monica wants to deceive Hilda. How to decide a preference? Nurse Evans was greatly troubled by this problem but decided that because Hilda has only a short time to live that the balance must be tipped in her favour.

As she thought about autonomy, and about what the expression might mean in a case such as this, Nurse Evans realised that both Hilda and Monica have unnecessarily limited autonomy. For instance, each is unaware of the other's feelings, and both lack certain pieces of relevant factual information which they might be made aware of. Nurse Evans pondered the box **create autonomy** – ought this to be the central inspiration for Dr Owens in this case?

With typical thoroughness Nurse Evans turned her attention to the black layer. As usual there were major uncertainties. How would Monica react if she knew her mother was dying? Would she feel differently about her mother going into a home? Nurse Evans put to one side the box **degree of certainty of the evidence on which action is taken**. Then she wondered if perhaps the problem was not essentially one of consequences. What might the consequences be if Dr Owens' promise to Hilda were to be broken? And what might the outcome be if it were explained to Hilda what a burden she was to her daughter in her sickness?

Nurse Evans studied the green layer. Is Dr Owens' priority the individual or the group – is her basic obligation to Hilda or to the whole family? She decided that the consultant could not make a reasonable, realistic decision thinking of Hilda in isolation. The box to select was surely **most beneficial outcome for a particular group**. She put this box to one side. Nurse Evans then reflected on the red layer, noted the importance of the boxes **tell the truth** and **keep promises**, but remembered that these principles may be overridden if a *greater degree of morality* will be attained by so doing (see p. 27). She took no box from this level because she considers **minimise harm** and **do most positive good** to be self-evident truths about health care.

Nurse Evans looked at the results of her survey of the Grid. She had extracted – but replaced – **respect autonomy**, since there appeared to be contradictory wishes. She was left with **create autonomy, degree of certainty of the evidence on which action is taken**, and **most beneficial outcome for a particular group**. In her opinion Dr Owens should break her promise to Hilda and tell Monica her mother is dying, and this is what she advises. In this way Hilda will have either the same or more control of the situation, and Monica will be able to make a more informed judgement. Monica will be enabled to review her decision about 'the home' in the light of her knowledge of her mother's illness – and so in addition may well avoid future regret and anguish.

Nurse Bryant

Nurse Bryant takes the view that a health worker's basic concern must always be for her patient. It is the patient who is ill, not the family as a rule, and it is the patient for whom doctors agree to care.

On studying the Grid Nurse Bryant was strongly attracted to the red level. Dr Owens has duties which conflict: should she **keep her promise** to Hilda, or should she **tell** Monica **the truth**? Two factors swayed Nurse Bryant's analysis. Firstly, she saw a difference between Hilda's request and Monica's. Hilda asked the doctor to withhold the truth from Monica (which in Nurse

Bryant's opinion is not the same as lying) but Monica has actually asked her to lie on her behalf. In truth Hilda is not so incapacitated that she must be permanently hospitalised. Secondly, and crucially, Hilda not Monica is the patient, and it is Hilda to whom Dr Owens has made her promise. In Nurse Bryant's eyes the doctor's responsibility is clear. She should keep her promise to Hilda. She should also speak to Monica and explain that she is not prepared to lie for her. She should suggest that Monica try to speak to Hilda about how hard it is for her to care for her mother, but it is not her job as a doctor to facilitate this process. Nurse Bryant carefully reviewed the rest of the Grid but was unable to shake off her perception of the importance of duty.

Dr Owens' decision

Dr Owens had not realised the implications of her promise to Hilda. For a time she was truly stuck about what to do, but, after sleeping on it, she decided that Nurse Bryant had the best solution, for the best reasons, in the long run. Hilda has a secret and wishes it to be kept. She is her patient while Monica is peripheral. It does not fall to her to overstep her clinical role. She is there to treat disease, injury and handicap to the best of her ability, not to become involved in family politics.

Discussion

This case raises many central issues in health care ethics: autonomy, utility, promise-keeping, and truth-telling. These factors are delicately balanced and might be arranged so as to sway Dr Owens one way or the other. However, the most effective way through the maze is to think in terms of *obligation*: if the doctor only has a duty to her patient the deliberation is relatively simple. If she has an obligation to the family it is more complicated, and if she thinks in terms of a duty to society it is harder still. There are complex resource implications both for the health service in general – and for Monica – resting on Dr Owens' decision. For example, ignoring any potential emotional complications and focusing only on practical consequences, to discharge Hilda reduces short-term cost to the hospital but may well increase the cost in terms of community care, and in long-term morbidity to both Monica and her child.

However, it remains true to say that the decision-making process becomes at least psychologically easier for the doctor the more simple she keeps her focus of care. It is obviously easier to decide what to do if Hilda is the only person whose wishes must be respected. Of course, this is not to say that the easiest option is the best. Never to consider the wider ramifications of one's decisions, and habitually to simplify complex situations in the same way, is the polar opposite of ethical deliberation. Such a mechanistic approach should be avoided for its own sake, because it adds nothing to the intellectual and caring capabilities of the doctor concerned, and because it often leads to bad practice.

EXERCISE

Reflect on the same case, but with one factor changed: Monica is a wealthy housewife, with a nine year old child, in a stable and happy marriage. Does this make any difference?

Advise Dr Owens with the help of the Grid.

Note: Maxine Bullen, at the time a student studying for Liverpool University's MSc in the Ethics of Health Care, provided the original material for this case study.

Case 5

A Duty to Society?

Introduction

The question of whether or not to keep secret information which has been conveyed in confidence is not only a dilemma for doctors. We have all, at one time or another, been placed in circumstances where we have to decide whether to reveal what we know to other people, or whether to keep quiet. Usually in such situations we consider telling the truth either because we believe that another person **ought** to know it (red), or because we believe that the other person will be **better off** because he knows the information (green). Most people will undertake a complex deliberation before arriving at a decision, although it will not be so ethically explicit as an analysis which uses the Grid or Algorithm.

Even though the question of whether or not to keep secrets is universal, the medical profession often finds itself at the centre of heated controversy over questions of confidentiality. On occasions it is true that the implications of keeping or breaking a confidence are more extensive in a medical context, but the ethical issues are basically the same as for any other person in possession of a secret. Neither the law nor the various codes of practice offer clear guidelines for doctors. Consequently ethical analysis is indispensable in such situations.

The Epileptic Driver

The situation

Dr Harrison is a GP whose patient, Mr Larkin, has developed epilepsy following a head injury. Mr Larkin is taking antiepileptic medication and has not had a fit for about six months. Mr Larkin knows that it is against the law for him to drive until he has been fit-free for two years, but he has nevertheless resumed doing so. Dr Harrison knows this both from Mrs Larkin, who originally approached him about her husband's behaviour, and from Mr Larkin himself, who says that he needs to drive in his new job. The doctor has explained to him that he ought not to drive and that doctors are expected to inform the DVLC of their epileptic patients. But Mr Larkin has shrugged off the warning. He has been unemployed several times in his life. Naturally his job means a lot to him and is essential for his family's financial well-being.

Dr Harrison is in a difficult position. What should he do? Should he contact the DVLC to inform them of Mr Larkin's behaviour? Or should he keep his silence and permit Mr Larkin to make his own choices?

The doctor's use of the Algorithm

Dr Harrison decides to make use of the Algorithm in order to ensure that he considers the problem as thoroughly as possible. Dr Harrison is drawn first to the quadrant Central Conditions of Health Work. He highlights two boxes as most important to this dilemma; these are **respect autonomy** and **respect persons equally**. But he sees that they conflict.

Mr Larkin wishes to be allowed to drive, but to permit this (in other words to **respect his autonomy**) will possibly endanger other drivers. In effect Larkin is asking for a form of positive discrimination which, if he were to be

Re: EPILEPSY :

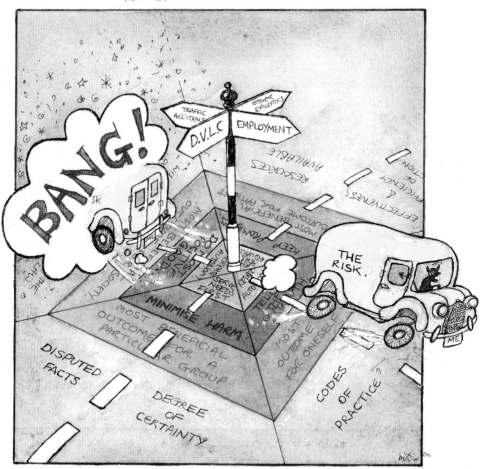

THE QUESTION OF ALLEGIANCE.

dispassionate, he might well find difficult to justify in a general context. Not to allow *anyone* with epilepsy to drive seems to be the only consistent policy of **equal respect**.

Dr Harrison needs to think more deeply and so continues to use the Algorithm.

He is **satisfied with the available information** but wonders what the medical justification is for the two-year ban on driving following a fit. Is there any hard evidence that after two years the risk of fitting is negligible, or is this ruling arbitrary? Statistically, what is the risk of having a fit after six months of being fit-free? Ought this level of risk to prohibit Mr Larkin driving? Dr Harrison calls a neurologist he knows for an authoritative opinion. The consultant satisfies him that on current medical knowledge the present limits are sensible. The risk of recurrence of seizures is approximately 10% per annum if on antiepileptic drugs and seizure-free for two years; the seizure risk at least doubles if the seizure-free time is halved to one year.[1]

The next part of the quadrant asks Dr Harrison to consider **the wishes of anyone else** involved in the case. Clearly the preferences of Mr Larkin's wife are important. She is worried about her husband's behaviour, and would rather have an unemployed husband than one in trouble with the law or, worse, dead. Consequently Dr Harrison notes Mrs Larkin's feelings and bears them in mind as he considers **the law** and **codes of practice**. The law is simply incontrovertible: anyone with a diagnosis of epilepsy should not drive a vehicle until fit-free for two years. The BMA code of practice[2] is more equivocal and says that a doctor 'like every other citizen, is a member of society with all the responsibilities this entails'. It goes on to say that when a conflict arises between a doctor's duty to society and duty of confidentiality then that doctor 'should seek to persuade the patient to disclose the information himself or give permission for the doctor to disclose it'. Dr Harrison has already tried to persuade Mr Larkin to stop driving and pointed out to him that it could be necessary for him to inform the DVLC if he continues to drive. In spite of this Mr Larkin has refused to promise to change his driving habits. The **code of practice** offers little further help to Dr Harrison. It simply says that it is 'for his conscience to decide on his further course of action'. So, still in doubt, Dr Harrison turns to the quadrant Moral Duties.

Of the four boxes available he picks **confidentiality** and **minimising harm** as priority duties, but does not think he can use them both at once. Firstly, he reasons that confidentiality is essential to the doctor/patient relationship. If patients do not feel that their doctors will maintain confidence then they will at best cease being fully open and honest in consultancy and at worst stop seeking help from the medical profession altogether. But then what if Mr Larkin fits whilst driving, thereby having a road accident and injuring both himself and others? Dr Harrison comes to the opinion that on balance **minimising harm** must, on this occasion, be ranked higher than the duty of **confidentiality**. After all, he thinks, there is no reason why his other patients should find out about this isolated failure to keep a confidence; besides, he can ultimately justify his choice in terms of an obligation to consider practical probabilities (so using the red and green parts of the Algorithm together). He must consider public safety, and he sees that he has chosen to rank his perceived duties with reference to likely outcomes.

Since he has been unable to think *purely* in terms of duty, the doctor moves into the final area of the Algorithm which addresses Consequences explicitly. If he does not act on the Larkins' information and omits to inform the DVLC he will please Mr Larkin in the short term but will this be to his patient's ultimate benefit? He reasons that, although Mr Larkin is at the moment happier employed as a driver than to be jobless, he could have an accident which might result in his injury or death. This outcome would certainly not benefit Mr Larkin or his family and seems to outweigh by far the current benefits of employment.

There may also be unwelcome consequences for Dr Harrison himself. If he decides not to inform Swansea things may be more comfortable for him personally; for instance, he will be spared a difficult, probably confrontational, interview with his patient. But in the end Dr Harrison decides that he will have to put up with this type of unpleasant consequence, and make his priority the protection of others. He recognises that if he does not, and an accident does happen, then there may be more severe and far-reaching consequences for all concerned.

At this stage he moves out of the Algorithm, since he thinks he has exhausted all its possibilities. He takes stock of his analysis, and studies the notes he has made. He observes that although he came to the conclusion that it is very important to **respect** Mr Larkin's **autonomy**, he also decided that the **consequences** of doing so could be detrimental to several parties. Moreover, he developed the view that his duty to **minimise harm** should take precedence over the duty to **keep confidences** in this situation.

His final judgement is that the weight of argument appears to support a decision to inform the DVLC of Mr Larkin's persistence in driving. The law would support this decision, and his professional code of practice does not counsel against it. So, despite the conflict between one Central Condition of Health Work and the conclusions drawn in the three other quadrants, Dr Harrison decides to inform the DVLC of his patient's condition.

EXERCISE

How might a different doctor, say a Dr Rautray, use the Algorithm to *justify* keeping Mr Larkin's confidence? Present the argument whether or not you agree with it.

References

1. A randomised study of antiepileptic drug withdrawal in patients in remission of epilepsy by the MRC Antiepileptic Drug Withdrawal Study Group. (1991) *Lancet*, 337:1175–80.
2. British Medical Association (1981) *The Handbook of Medical Ethics*, p. 13, section 1.11. London: BMA.

Case 6

Communication

Introduction

Although not essentially a *clinical* skill most medical activity involves communication of some kind. Communication between doctor and patient is a particularly central feature of general practice. The patient must be able to describe his symptoms in a way which will not mislead the doctor, while the GP must be able to explain his proposed treatment and what effects the patient might anticipate. Beyond this there is significant dispute about what should count as desirable, and what ought to be considered effective doctor/patient communication. Some doctors prefer to restrict themselves to communicating the barest minimum information they believe the patient needs to know, while others advocate a policy of complete openness. The latter type of doctor will often discuss notes and records with the patient, checking that he or she is happy they are accurate. And, rather than pretend to have absolutely authoritative knowledge about diagnosis and treatment, this sort of doctor will share his thoughts and uncertainties with the patient.

The first model of doctor – the doctor as complete expert, the 'paternalistic' doctor – has been roundly criticised by very many writers over the last three decades. The most significant objections to this form of practice have been that patients have a basic right to understand what is happening, or is to happen, to their bodies; that the choice about what to do for a patient ought ultimately to be made by the patient rather than the doctor; and that the role of the doctor is not merely to instruct a person about how to take tablets or undertake a particular therapy, but to educate patients in a broader fashion.[1,2]

On the other hand, critics of the 'open doctor' model point out that, however much she might wish to be honest and to share information with patients, certain uncomfortable facts remain. Firstly, the patient, not the doctor, is the one with the problem. Not only does this make the patient more vulnerable, but it also means that the complaint is more important to her than it is to the doctor. So 'sharing' is not, and cannot be, a perfectly balanced equation. Secondly, the doctor, not the patient, has specialist medical knowledge, as well as the power to prescribe treatment. Once again, there is a pronounced imbalance. Consequently, it is argued, the idea of a free and open consultation owes more to wishful thinking on the part of liberal doctors than it does to an examination of the facts. In addition it is argued that not all patients *wish* to 'share' decision making. Their reason for approaching a doctor is to take advantage of expert knowledge which has taken a long time to acquire. Some patients realise that they can never hope to attain a useful understanding of the complexities of their clinical problem. Consequently a proportion of patients are happy for the 'expert doctor' to take responsibility for decision making. They want to feel confident in their doctors, and can be alarmed by doctors who have deliberately dismantled their air of authority.

The debate between these two schools goes on. However, as the following case demonstrates, at least it is certain that issues of communication always have significant ethical content. Neither of the doctors involved in the conversation described below make use of the Grid or Algorithm. However, occasions where they raise the various ethical categories are indicated. The doctors do not necessarily wish to assert the category in question, but each is noted, in either bold or italic type, to show the ethical focus of their discussion.

The Ideal Communication?

The situation

Dr Peterson is feeling pleased with himself. He has been commissioned by the Royal Society of Medicine to produce a video series called *Doctor/Patient Conversations*, and has just completed the fourth tape (out of six). This video is meant to show a trouble-free encounter – Programme Four is to offer a model of good practice.

Dr Peterson is proud of his ability to communicate sensitively with his patients, whilst at the same time diagnosing and prescribing efficiently, and within a reasonable time limit. He has videoed, with the patients' permission, an entire weeks' consultations. On reviewing his films he believes that he has come up with a 'gem'.

He thinks his best video records a meeting with Mary. She is 27 years old, 32 weeks pregnant, and an asthmatic. Mary has found that her asthma has been worsening as her pregnancy developed. Consequently she made an appointment with Dr Peterson. From Mary's perspective this appointment was made not to *discuss* her condition, but in order for her to make a specific request of the doctor. From Dr Peterson's perspective the consultation was to be an 'open conversation' about the best way to manage the patient's condition.

Mary has been asthmatic since birth. She was diagnosed at eight months and all her life has had to cope with a disabling and sometimes terrifying condition. Mary is, as she says, an expert about *her* asthma.

Mary already has a child of 18 months. During her first pregnancy she experienced difficulty with breathing. However, for almost the entire nine months she was able to control her asthma effectively by use of a nebuliser (a piece of electrical equipment which costs approximately £100 and dispenses drugs in droplet form by mask) which delivered salbutamol in droplet form. Salbutamol is a bronchodilator used to dilate narrowed tubes. However, salbutamol acts only on the 'spasm' element of asthma. The more serious 'inflammation' element of the condition – when the lining of the tubes swells and fluid collects – is treated by steroids. Long-term steroid treatment is given by inhaler, short-term by a course of tablets to be taken orally. Steroids taken by mouth can cause weight gain, high blood pressure or both. In pregnancy they might cause the baby to be heavier than he might otherwise have been, but this is not necessarily a problem. Any side-effects ought to be negligible with a one-week course.

Mary does not want steroids because she is afraid of the effect on her unborn child. Towards the end of her previous pregnancy she was persuaded to take steroids. But when the baby was born it cried non-stop for two days, a problem which she attributed to her steroid therapy. Mary would again like to take salbutamol by nebuliser. This method is highly efficient, but there is danger of overdosing, and that the nebuliser may make the patient feel better but disguise truly worsening asthma. For this reason doctors prefer to supervise the use of nebulisers. Dr Peterson's clear preference in any case of this kind is to prescribe a seven-day course of steroids to be taken orally.

Dr Peterson plays his video to Dr Smail, who is co-producer of the series. To Peterson's surprise Smail does not seem particularly impressed.

'I thought you said this is a classic Alan.'

'Yes. Surely this is as close to the perfect consultation as you can get,' responds Peterson defensively. 'I was kind but forceful, I explained to Mary that oral steroids for seven days would be the *most effective treatment*, I told her there was nothing to worry about with the oral steroids – the *fact* that her other child cried for two days after birth was *not due* to steroids. I checked the progress of the pregnancy, I tried to find if Mary had any other worries she wanted to tell me, and she went away – happy, yes I believe she was happy – with a prescription for her asthma. What more could I do?'

'Well,' Smail continues. 'I don't think that's the only way it could've gone. Let's go over precisely what happened, and then you can try to justify what you did. I'll listen and then I'll criticise you – constructively, as we agreed – and suggest an alternative.'

'Okay. You're on. I'd like to hear what you would've done instead.'

Smail and Peterson watch a re-run of the video. Peterson, still satisfied with his performance, sits back and allows his colleague to stop the film from time to time, and to comment. As the video begins Tony Smail checks, 'We both know the circumstances of the patient, and the basic clinical facts. Yes? Fine, then let's look at what you did step by step.'

Smail stops the video. 'Look at that. Now Mary is clearly anxious as she enters, but looks very determined too. You ask what the problem is and she delivers an obviously prepared speech. Her asthma scares her – especially when she can neither breathe nor talk – she's used a nebuliser before during pregnancy – she doesn't want oral steroids because it could make baby podgy – she doesn't want drugs in her bloodstream; better in her lungs.'

'Of course she is just offering a lay-person's perception. You know that if her attacks are so bad then a short course of steroids by mouth is the answer, whatever she thinks.'

'Yes, that's probably true, but in my opinion you *haven't taken proper account of her anxieties* (**serve needs first**),' says Smail. 'Let's run it on . . . Look, here she says that

Re: COMMUNICATION:

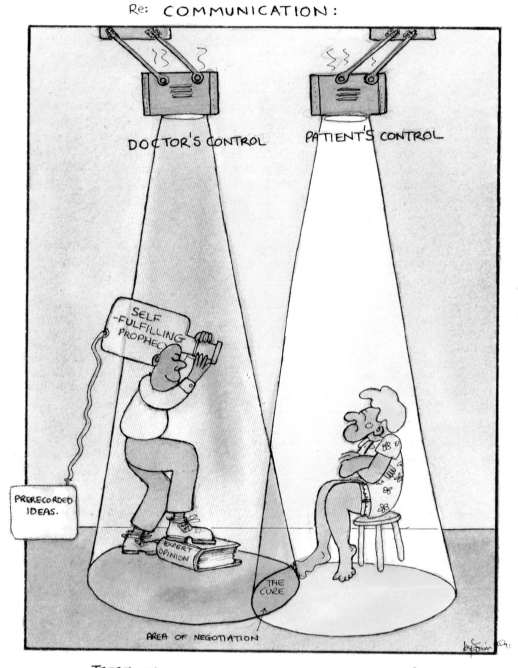

TREATMENT BY IMPOSITION OR NEGOTIATION?

Dr Brough, from the asthma clinic, said that if she was told she needed steroids again she was to contact him for a nebuliser. But you seem to shrug off this idea. Steroids are the thing, and its pretty clear to me – and to her come to that – that steroids are the only treatment she's going to come away with . . . Now, she's trying for the last time with you – she was *very* sensible last time she used a nebuliser, she even had to tell the nurses in the maternity ward how to use it. She's not coming out with it specifically, but she's saying to you that you don't trust her – she knows her body, *she knows what she wants* (**respect autonomy**), but you won't give it to her. What's more, Alan, I don't think that you are really *explaining* anything to her (**create autonomy**) – all you are doing is stating that steroids are best and that patients must be careful when using nebulisers. I don't think she's happy at all, and I think – though I haven't examined her – that a nebuliser would see her through to term, and then she *will become less anxious* too (**disputed facts**). Sorry, I've told you what I think now – but you don't agree?'

'No I don't,' Alan replies, a little angry, but controlled and articulate. 'Perhaps it is not the best communication in the world but outside I had *a waiting room full* of coughs, colds, screaming kids – and some serious illness too (**wishes of others**). I did not have the time to explain the pharmacological properties of corticosteroids. I did *explain* that they would control asthma without affecting her weight unduly, and that the baby could not be harmed (**tell the truth, create autonomy**). And, you should know, when she took the steroids *her condition rapidly improved and her chest was clear three days later.*'

'But that's not the main point Alan. Basically you patronised her. You said – doctor knows best, nebulisers shouldn't be toyed with, your fears are exaggerated, take the medicine. I bet you that she has little understanding, or even totally the wrong message, about why you wanted her to take steroids. You made up her mind for her. Any discussion you had was just superficial.'

Alan speaks after thinking for a few seconds. 'Alright, your interpretation might be correct, maybe I was telling her what to do. But *that's what I'm here for.* It is not my place *to tell Mary everything* there is to know about asthma therapy (**truth-telling**). My job is to manage her clinical condition, tell her what she needs to know, and *help her as quickly as possible* (**most beneficial outcome for the patient**). The doctor/patient communication is not a casual conversation but a structured one, it is a vehicle for *instruction* – the patient instructs me about how she feels – *I instruct her* about what's best to do (**create autonomy**). I give her my advice and the benefit of my experience, and I expect her to take it.'

Discussion

Basically Dr Peterson's argument rests on an appeal to duty and consequences. In his opinion the purpose of medicine is not for doctors to communicate on equal terms with patients, but to make sure that they receive the best possible clinical therapy. That is the clinical responsibility (red) – and the test is the success or failure of the treatment (green). Mary's treatment was a success, everything she needed to know was told to her, therefore the whole episode should be classified as a model encounter.

Dr Smail agrees with his partner that the treatment prescribed was the best clinical option, but he does not think that it was the only option. Perhaps the bronchodilator would have been less effective, but it would still have afforded Mary some relief, and certainly less anxiety. Dr Smail does not think that medicine is such an automated enterprise that every decision must be driven entirely by clinical criteria and priorities. Caring doctors should take account of their patients' wants – even if these wishes are not based on the same premises or pattern of reasoning the doctor would use. Not to do this is not respectful, and can cause anxiety, stress and unhappiness. Medicine, if it is to have any real value, must be humane.

EXERCISE

1. Review any one of the consultations in which you have been involved during the last week and try to explain your actions in the terms of the Ethical Grid.

2. Consider how you might have handled the consultation differently and explain this using the Grid's categories.

If you are a medical student then reflect upon any consultations you have witnessed or, failing that, consider consultations where you have been the patient, and attempt the two exercises from the perspective of the doctor.

References

1. Kennedy, I. (1981) *The Unmasking of Medicine*. London: Penguin.
2. Seedhouse, D.F. (1986) *Health: The Foundations for Achievement*. Chichester: John Wiley and Sons.

Case 7

Informed Consent

Introduction

This case reveals the reasoning process undertaken by a surgeon who is deliberating about how much information it is appropriate to give to a patient. He is guided in his thinking by the Algorithm. Naturally questions about information and consent are not asked only by surgeons. On the contrary, the issue is of great relevance to most doctors. Many substantial ethical puzzles continue to surround the topic, and the issue has also generated extensive commentary in legal circles.

The scenario presented below describes an attempted justification of a policy not to tell a patient of a particular risk factor in an operation. The analyses have general implications for all situations in which doctors must decide how much they should reveal to patients. In theory it is possible to hold one of two quite simple views about the disclosure of risk: either that it should be up to the doctor, as a professional expert, to decide how much to tell – and if he decides to tell nothing then that is acceptable; or that absolutely every possible risk should be conveyed to the patient – in other words that 'the whole truth' should be told whatever the doctor thinks. However, neither position is realistic. The first is of dubious morality, particularly if a person is given no information at all. In such circumstances he cannot possibly make an informed judgement about what is to happen to him, and any intervention made cannot, strictly speaking, be lawful since competent patients must at least have a 'general understanding' of the nature of the intended operation or procedure. The second position raises an important question about the meaning of 'the truth' in such cases. If the expression 'the whole truth' is taken literally then it could be argued that a doctor ought to explain every possible risk, however minor, and should also ensure that the patient has the fullest possible understanding of the clinical background to the proposed procedure. But such a policy is clearly impracticable.

In reality the doctor must steer a path between the two poles. This is done routinely by very many clinicians. But just because the process of judgement is done frequently this does not necessarily mean that it is always done as well as possible. It is one thing to follow an established course of action because it has been successful, or at least not challenged, yet it can be quite another to explain to others *why* the policy is the most appropriate possible.

Clinical Licence?

The situation

Mr Aziz considers himself to be an efficient and caring surgeon. He has a clear policy that he will never delegate the task of discussing a forthcoming operation. He is always busy but insists on explaining the essential aspects of the proposed operation to each patient. His minimum requirement is that each patient is aware that there is some risk during any surgical procedure.

Recently Mr Walker, a contemporary of Aziz's at medical school, has only narrowly avoided legal action in negligence for not revealing a 'significant risk' to a patient. Mr Walker would probably have been sued if it were not for the potentially huge financial cost to the plaintiff (who was not entitled to legal aid) were the action to prove unsuccessful. The two doctors met to discuss the case. Mr Walker outlined the general situation, and explained the nub of the patient's grievance as he understood it from a lengthy letter from her solicitor.

Walker began, 'Mrs Cullen is a 40 year old woman of nervous disposition; she was admitted for a routine cholecystectomy following the failure of more conservative methods of treatment. The operation was successful but she developed deep vein thrombosis (DVT) shortly afterwards. This meant that she had to stay in hospital for somewhat longer than anticipated, unfortunately in considerable discomfort. Mrs Cullen claimed, she says truthfully, that I did not tell her about this complication and if I had then she would not have consented to the operation. I don't think that I should have told her because this might have upset her, and prevented the useful operation. Also, the risk of a DVT is low, as you know.

'I must say I was surprised at how upset Mrs Cullen was. She said – at least she said through the pen of her lawyer – that I had robbed her of an autonomous choice. How could she make an informed decision about whether to have the operation when not in possession of all the facts?

'She also accused me of arrogance, and insufficient attention to evidence. She said that I have very little information about herself and her family, but nevertheless jumped to conclusions about her psychological stability and ability to make objective decisions. I think she was quite unfair here since we actually have comprehensive medical records on her.

'She claims that her faith in doctors has been broken. She cannot see how my "god-like" approach can be good for other patients. Her argument is that no doctor ought to shoulder total responsibility for decisions about patient care. Indeed, in her opinion the community as a whole will suffer if its members are prevented from making decisions for themselves.

'Now I think that a lot of this is hysterical, particularly where she insists that she is not a child, but the threat of action has caused me to think about policy. We've always had a similar style and approach. Tell me, if you were asked to justify not telling Mrs Cullen – or Mrs Smith or Mrs Brown or Mrs Jones – about the risk of DVT, how would you go about it?'

Mr Aziz's reply was based on a step by step, steady analysis. He began, 'I would use the Algorithm here. As you know there are four quadrants to the

Algorithm and I can enter at any one of these. Like you I am a practical man, so I would begin by thinking about Consequences. I have a choice of four boxes here. Dependent upon which I decide to emphasise, my justification may be different. First I need to resolve my priority. Am I most concerned to increase **benefit** for the patient, for her family and friends, for myself, or for society? Well, this is not difficult for a doctor. Of course my priority must be my patient – I must ensure that I apply my clinical skills to maximise her health status. I know that she's nervous, and I know she requires the operation, so I think the calculation is straightforward.

'My position is reinforced as I move into the Central Conditions of Health Work quadrant. There are two relevant boxes here: **create autonomy** and **serve needs first**. By operating I add to her health and give her more control – so I create autonomy in the patient. And of course I serve a fundamental need.'

'But,' Mr Walker interrupted, 'wouldn't she say that you should have selected the other two available boxes: **respect autonomy** and **respect persons equally**? In reality the patient claimed that she did not have sufficient choice. Surely she would say to you that you should have told her more, so respecting her capacity to choose. She might also have argued that if you'd been operating on me, or a nurse, then you would've explained much more about the risks.'

'Agreed. But I am offering *my* justification and I cannot use all the boxes at once because they conflict.

'The next quadrant is easier though. I would be, as you were, **satisfied with the available information** and naturally I would be pursuing the proper medical course of action. No-one else's **wishes** are relevant here since I have already decided that it is the patient who must be the priority. I would be acting in the best interest of Mrs Cullen and so I would be abiding by our **code of practice**. **The law** may be another matter, but I rather think that as a responsible and reasonable man I would be well supported by my professional colleagues.

'The remaining quadrant refers to Duty. It would be fair to say that by not telling Mrs Cullen of the risk of DVT that I would not be one hundred percent honest – although if she asked me outright "Will I suffer a DVT?", or words to that effect, then I would not lie. However, I would choose **doing positive good** and **minimising harm** before the putative duty to **tell the truth**. If she has the operation she will be able to return to a far richer, more fulfilling life, and I would not have caused her any unnecessary anxiety by worrying her about an unlikely risk. We must remember that most patients do not suffer DVTs, and that we can only judge what to do prior to the operation. It is only judges, solicitors, and philosophers who exploit the advantage of hindsight.'

EXERCISE

Whether you agree with Mrs Cullen and her solicitor or not, use the Algorithm to elaborate on her counter-position, and to challenge the doctors.

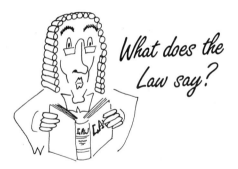

What does the Law say?

It is not practicable in a casebook of this size to undertake complex analysis of any kind. Case 11 begins to indicate the depth at which the most thorough *ethical analysis* can be undertaken.

Legal analysis is, if anything, even more puzzling to non-lawyers than ethics since judges do not argue directly from ethical principles but from a complicated and controversial mix of legal precedent. Consent is a particularly factious subject area. To give something of the flavour of the legal debate the following edited extract from an ethics thesis is helpful:

The English Legal Position

Margaret Brazier writes in *Medicine, Patients and the Law*[1] that 'every adult has an inviolable right to determine what is done to his or her own body' (p. 55). However, it is far from certain that this principle is reflected in English case law relating to consent. Although there has been some broadening of the legal concept of consent over the last fifty years, real changes seem to have been minimal. The English legal notion of consent is still very much a narrow one.

Consent

Any consideration of the English legal notion of consent must begin with the 1957 case of *Bolam v McFriern H.M.C.* It was held that the relevant test (of negligence or not) for a surgeon was that of 'the ordinary skilled man exercising and professing to have that special skill'. McNair J. also argued that where there was more than one 'proper standard', this had no bearing on the case as long as the doctor followed 'a practice accepted as proper by a responsible body of medical men skilled in that particular art' (121, c-122 b). This means that the degree of information given to a patient, like matters of diagnosis and treatment, are decided by the medical profession itself. This was an improvement upon Denning's judgement in *Hatcher v Black* (1954) which suggested a *subjective* professional judgement, where it appeared a doctor could withhold information because he felt it was necessary to do so, regardless of what other doctors might think. *Bolam* has been approved in a succession of relevant cases, most notably, at all levels, in *Sidaway v Bethlem Royal Hospital Governors* (1985).

Sidaway was taken to the House of Lords to clarify that the *Bolam* test
continued

continued

applied to advice as well as diagnosis and treatment. The majority decision appears to be that it clearly did. Lord Diplock was the most forceful when he argued that,

> 'to decide what risks the existence of which a patient should be voluntarily warned and the terms in which such warning, if any, should be given, having regard to the effect that the warning may have, is as much an exercise of professional skill and judgement as any other part of the doctor's comprehensive duty of care to the individual patient, and expert medical evidence on this matter should be treated in just the same way. The *Bolam* test should be applied.'

It was held by all the Lords, except by Diplock who would undoubtedly agree although he did not mention it, that a doctor may be fulfilling his duty to care even if he withholds information, on the grounds that it may be damaging to that patient. Lord Bridge warned of the danger that a patient, on receiving information of a risk,

> 'even though [the doctor] describes it as remote, may lead to that risk assuming an undue significance in the patient's calculations.'

Lord Templeman argued that a doctor is under a specific duty to withhold information where in the doctor's opinion it may harm the patient. Information given must be, 'subject always to the doctor's own obligation to say and do nothing which the doctor is satisfied will be harmful to the patient'. Lord Scarman agreed that there needed to be an element of what he termed 'therapeutic privilege'. Skegg goes so far as to suggest that a doctor may be liable if information which he gave was shown to have caused a patient harm. He cites the New Zealand case of *Furniss v Fitchett* (1958). In English law this remains an unexplored, but very real, possibility.

The only new legal principle which can safely be derived from *Sidaway* is that when asked specific questions a doctor must not withhold or conceal information. It looks as though part of a doctor's duty of care is to answer questions put to him by a patient truthfully, and as fully as required; otherwise he may be found negligent. However, since this ruling there seems to have been little change in respect of a plaintiff sueing successfully.

Dawson, A., Unit for the Study of Health Care Ethics, Liverpool University.

Reference

1. Brazier, M. (1987) *Medicine, Patients and the Law*. London: Penguin.

Note: There is a 10–20% risk of DVT following a cholecystectomy, but only 4–5% are clinically apparent. However, these figures are for patients who have not been on a prophylactic such as heparin, and this therapy is routine. *BJ Hosp Med*, 1988, vol. 40, p. 146.

Case 8

Truth Hurts?

Background

Mrs Theresa Hennessey, 67, presented with a cough and weight loss. Her husband had died 15 years earlier of lung cancer and she feared that she had the same problem. Her GP referred her to the local hospital where, following X-rays showing a shadow, a bronchoscopy and biopsy was performed which confirmed a diagnosis of lung cancer. Further tests showed she had metastases in her liver and brain, and so surgery was not performed.

Mrs Hennessey was told of her lung cancer. It was also explained to her that her condition was now inoperable, but that irradiation treatment could be helpful. Doctors met with Mrs Hennessey's close family – her twin sister, her three adult children and her sister-in-law. They explained the full picture. The consultant described Mrs Hennessey's prognosis as 'extremely bleak' and said she would not have long to live. The shocked family agreed that it would be best not to tell Theresa the extent of her cancer.

Mrs Hennessey soon developed headaches and visual disturbance which she put down to the irradiation therapy. Although these symptoms alarmed her she did not specifically ask the doctor their cause. After a month of irradiation treatment, she became so weak that her doctors felt this treatment ought to be withdrawn, although they increased her pain relief since her headaches were severe. Mrs Hennessey died five days later. Until the end her family, and the hospital staff, remained encouraging. She was never aware of the extent of her cancer, although she knew she was dying.

Like all the cases in this book this one is real and is far from uncommon. It is more subtle than the usual 'medical ethics' truth-telling case since the patient knew much of what was wrong with her, but she did not know it all. It raises several ethical issues – some of which are discussed in the ethics class described below. One is especially interesting: *is there such a thing as an 'emotional pain threshold', can we know it, and do doctors have any special right to assess whether or not it should be crossed?*

The Ethics Class

Months after Mrs Hennessey's death a class of medical students discussed her case. The group's task was to reach an answer to the following question: did the medical intervention in the lives of Mrs Hennessey and her relatives achieve the *highest degree of morality* (see p. 27) – in other words, was it the best possible? Their supplementary question was: if it was not, how should the consultant have acted differently? Three of the student responses are reported below. References to aspects of the Grid and Algorithm are indicated by the appropriate colour in parentheses.

David

'I take the view that the doctor was *absolutely right* in this case. Yes, the highest degree of morality was definitely achieved. Mrs Hennessey knew that she had inoperable cancer, she knew that everything possible was being done for her, and she had the full care and support of her family – who did know the whole truth. What was to be gained by telling Mrs Hennessey that she had carcinomas in other parts of her body as well (green)? I've seen a few cancer patients now and, obviously . . . they find their condition very hard to come to terms with. You know, some of them actually feel guilty. They feel that they have somehow been weak, they've failed, they've let everybody down. To tell someone that she's riddled with cancer simply cannot make anything any better for anyone. I think that doctors have an elementary duty in these cases. They have to deal with suffering of many kinds – physical, emotional, spiritual and social – and in every case they are charged with the task to reduce harm wherever possible (red). This they did, and with great skill and care apparently. There was nothing more medically which they could have done; they relieved physical pain to an optimum level, they reassured the patient, and they made sure that she was always surrounded by people who loved her. There's no need to address the supplementary question.'

Elizabeth

'I agree with that analysis, although I would place the ethical emphasis differently. Yes, doctors should always do as little harm as possible (red), but this is not the key factor here. There are three other factors that I think are crucial: the risk (black), the need (blue), and respect for autonomy (blue). You have to remember why the medical profession exists. It isn't first of all to counsel or to educate patients; it is to carry out clinical work, in the interest of the patient, as efficiently as possible. The patient had a medical need (blue) for treatment for her widespread cancer. To deliver this treatment must be the medical priority. Now, if she were to have been told about the metastases, there would have been a significant risk (black) that she would have refused treatment and given up. Okay, I know that someone's going to say "she ought to have been given the choice", but the answer to that is that she *did* have the choice to refuse treatment in any case. The reason she wasn't told the entire truth was to prevent further harm (red and green) to her emotional condition. It must be hard to think straight anyway when you know you have cancer, but who can make a rational decision when they're told that their body's rotten? And you must bear in mind the basic duty to respect autonomy (blue).

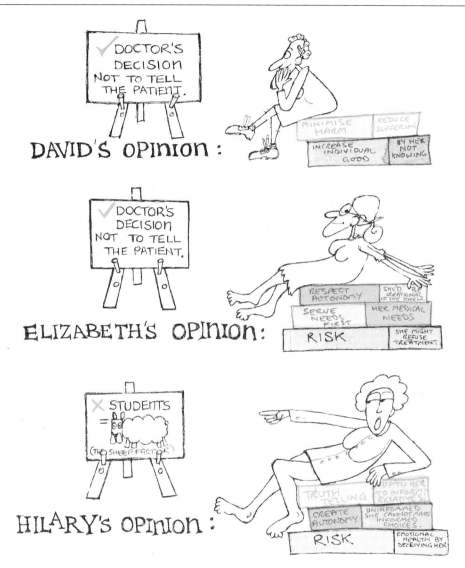

The patient's family was told absolutely everything, and they decided that she should be protected. If the doctors had gone against the family's wishes (black) then that would have been a different matter. But what happened was best for everybody.'

Hilary

'I suppose those are both reasonable arguments. But I've heard them before – over and over again. They are heard in every ward in this hospital. It's part of the "sheep factor", isn't it? Medical students get into medical schools because we absorb facts well and because we do what we're told to do. As a result young doctors slot quickly into the system. We learn rules quickly, we learn not to rock the boat, and – which really scares me – we continue to "soak up" what to think right down the line. We don't work it out for ourselves. The two previous speakers just parroted what they've picked up. Like buckets you fill them up, tip them up, and out it comes just like it went in. It's like there's no alternative, but of course there is.

'I think that what happened to Mrs Hennessey was appalling. I don't mean that she wasn't treated properly in a clinical sense, but she *was* abused. A 67 year old lady, and she was treated like a child where everyone else decided what she should know, leaving her to wonder, frightened, *entirely on her own*. What do you think it feels like to know that you are dying while everyone else is to go on living, and they're standing over your bed not knowing what to say, or crying, or generally behaving as if everything will be alright? And all the time they know the truth – truth about you, your truth, nobody else's.

'Perhaps she didn't know that everyone else was in on the secret of her metastases, perhaps she did. What if she did? What about the risk (black) to her "emotional health" then? And if she was being deceived, which is undeniable however much you twist the meaning of words, then how could she really choose (blue) whether to have chemotherapy and radiotherapy? Perhaps with a single growth she might think there's a chance? But with several secondaries? Is it worth the vomiting and the baldness then?

'I don't think that the purpose of medicine is primarily to be clinically efficient. I think we're here to work for health, and that basically means empowering the patients. Not just giving them power to fight disease but to give them power to decide what best to do with whatever life they have (blue). This is what is so distressing about Mrs Hennessey. She was told a lot but she still had a false view of her options. The doctors took over. The doctors took charge of life. Mrs Hennessey should have been told the truth (red) and then it would have been for her to tell her relatives, *if she wanted to*. Did anybody trouble to ask her whether she liked her relatives? Did they really care for her?

'What really gets me about this is the culture of secrecy. It's not just medicine, it seems to plague the whole country. Why is it that we cannot bring ourselves to tell the truth? Why is it so unsettling to us? What is better about deceit, particularly in terminal illness, when the facts will inevitably overtake us? When I qualify my policy will be, on every occasion, to tell the whole truth to every patient (blue and red), whether they say they want to hear it or not. Everybody has a basic need to know (blue), even though they might sometimes deny this psychologically.

'To answer the two questions directly: no, the highest degree of morality was not achieved by the consultant's intervention. It wasn't totally immoral, but it could've been a lot better, a lot kinder, a lot more respectful. Mrs Hennessey ought to have been told, whatever the perceived risk to her "emotional health" – to be in ignorance means that you can't have "emotional health" anyway.'

EXERCISE

Which student's position do you find most convincing? How would you add further strength to that position? Which aspects of the position cause you disquet? Which aspects of the alternative position(s) worry you?

Refer to the categories of either the Ethical Grid or the Algorithm in your answer.

Case 9

Screening

Introduction

Questions over the value of screening are of huge ethical import. Arguably they are significantly more far reaching than any other ethical question in health care, including those over embryo research, euthanasia and abortion. The recent changes in screening policy in the NHS[1] touch most of us in one way or another yet arouse little interest in 'medical ethics' circles. Perhaps one reason for this is that screening is such a massive operation, with consequences for the majority of professionals within the health service, that it is simply thought of as 'part of the job'. And to those accustomed to conceiving of ethical issues as discrete, occasional problems, it is hard to see how screening could be categorised as an 'ethical issue'. However, by now students of this casebook will be under no such misapprehension.

The issues

In 1990 changes in the GP contract compelled GPs to undertake certain screening procedures on patients. Doctors are required to offer a 'health check' once every three years to all patients between 16 and 74. Patients have to be invited to the surgery, where a history must be taken, as well as a brief examination which includes a check on blood pressure, height and weight, allergies, lifestyle problems (smoking, drinking, exercise), and social problems. GPs are also contractually obliged to see (either in the surgery or at home) all patients of 75 and over once a year whether they are regular patients or not. Checks for this group include social problems, ambulatory ability, urine testing (for glucose), and blood pressure.

Although not a direct compulsion, doctors are offered strong incentives to meet other screening targets. Some might argue that the level of incentive virtually creates compulsion. For example, the top target for cervical screening is 80% of the defined population. For this a doctor can expect £2,202 (January 1991 figure), but if he achieves only 50% and above (but not 80%) he will receive £734. Thus, nearly £1,500 can be at stake, and can rest on the consent of a single patient.

It is commonly said that the basic purposes of screening are to reduce preventable morbidity and mortality, and to save the NHS money. On the face of it, it is hard to see how anyone might object to screening since it seems to offer the opportunity to diagnose medical troubles early (perhaps even before a condition becomes problematic), and to treat with the greatest effectiveness and at the lowest possible financial cost. However, it is not so simple.

In a recent paper in the *British Medical Journal* Mant and Fowler[1] point out:

> '*The Need for Caution*
>
> Screening has the potential to do more harm than good. In the 1950s considerable enthusiasm was engendered for mass radiography and sputum cytology as screening tests for lung cancer. At first, screening seemed to offer great benefit: in one of the largest population based screening studies the proportion of cancers detected sufficiently early to be treated with surgery was almost 50%, and the five year survival was 35% – more than twice that in the control population. It was therefore a great disappointment that 10 years after screening began the cumulative mortality from lung cancer was identical in the screened and control populations.
>
> The experience of lung cancer screening should be remembered by those who try to justify screening in terms of high yields of disease, early stage at diagnosis, or even improved survival. Screening always advances diagnosis (the "lead time") and thereby improves survival from the time of diagnosis, but not necessarily from the time when the patient would have presented clinically. This is why screening is beguiling, and comparison of overall mortality and morbidity must be the final arbiter of efficacy.'

The authors go on to say that in the general enthusiasm for prevention rather than cure screening is often promoted without appropriate consideration of its efficacy or practical feasibility. However, there is good evidence that cervical cytology and mammography 'will save lives if properly organised'. In order to help ensure this, Mant and Fowler suggest 'minimum criteria' for mass screening in general practice. They suggest that before screening anyone, general practitioners should have answered these questions to their satisfaction:

- Can we offer effective treatment for patients positive on testing?
- How many positive tests will prove to be false alarms (and is this acceptable)?
- How many patients will need follow up over the next five years (and can we sustain this workload)?
- How are we going to audit routinely the quality of the test, of the intervention, and of follow up?

If doctors are not entirely satisfied with their answers to these questions they may need to conduct an ethical analysis of their practice. Doctors will have to consider a number of issues, all of which they will be reminded of if they consult the Ethical Grid. We will focus on one level at a time.

The black level (in particular: disputed facts, the degree of certainty of the evidence on which action is taken)

It is by no means certain beyond reasonable doubt that earlier detection means more effective treatment; there is a considerable difficulty over the appearance of 'false positives' in screening, and uncertainty about the predictive value of tests:

'Assessing the test: false positives and false negatives

Screening tests are traditionally described in terms of their sensitivity and specificity. Essentially a 'sensitive' test is one that rarely misses diseases, whereas a 'specific' test causes few false alarms.* The concepts of sensitivity and specificity are used to characterise a screening test because they do not depend on the setting in which the test is carried out. Sensitivity is assessed on patients with disease; specificity is assessed on healthy individuals. However, in the clinical setting a screening test is applied to a mixture of people with and without disease. At this stage the practitioner is interested in the number of patients who have positive test results (for these must be followed up and further investigated) and in the number of false alarms. The proportion of patients with positive results who actually have the disease is termed the positive predictive value of the test.

The predictive value . . . varies greatly in different settings . . . A test (or clinical symptom or sign) may give a high predictive value in a hospital setting but may be of very little value in the community. Misunderstanding of this important point will lead to inappropriate screening and unfounded criticism of general practitioners by their hospital colleagues.'

The green level

The assessment of the relationship between benefit and harm in screening is an intensely difficult one. Some people (although the proportion is not clear) will benefit from screening in that they will be spared a particular disease. Against this the doctor has to take the various costs of screening into account. These costs are of different types. Some are easy to measure and some practically impossible. Equally it is notoriously difficult, and distasteful to many, to balance the following types of costs against a human life saved:

'Costs of screening

Costs to the patients

- Economic loss (lost work, increased insurance premiums)
- False reassurance to some patients
- Unnecessary anxiety and further investigation for some patients
- Psychological harm

Costs to the practice

- Time and resource cost of test
- Time and resource cost of follow up

---

*Although a 'sensitive' test rarely misses disease it can give rise to a number of false positive results. A 'specific' test, on the other hand, gives a minimum risk of false positives, but at the cost that some patients with disease will be missed (false negatives). There is a fine balance to be struck between sensitivity and specificity for a screening test.

Costs to the NHS

- Reimbursements to practice from "Family Practitioner Committee"*
- Prescribing costs
- Increased use of hospital facilities.'

Mant and Fowler elaborate:

'Outcome of screening: costs and benefits

The costs and benefits of screening are extremely difficult to quantify. Benefits are most easily measured in terms of improvement in morbidity and mortality, and when possible these must be established by randomised trial. There may also be a long term benefit to the health service in terms of future treatment avoided.

Economic costs are no easier to establish than personal costs. For the general practitioner it is usually the marginal cost of the test (for example, the urine dipstick) and of the follow up time that must be weighed against payments from the Family Practitioner Committee. For the health service as a whole the average cost is more important, and the capital costs of building as well as of investigations and long term treatment must be considered. Analyses have been carried out to try to establish the cost-benefit ratio for screening. For example, it was calculated in 1985 that 40,000 smears and 200 excision biopsies were being carried out in Britain to prevent one death from cervical cancer. Figures given for the cost per life saved have been as high as £300,000 for cervical screening.'

The red level (in particular: minimise harm, tell the truth)

A GP may consider that she has a duty to **minimise harm** – but in order to perform this duty she has to be clear about precisely which harm or harms she wishes to keep to a minimum. Does she assess the worth of her practice in terms of comparative morbidity and mortality figures with other practices? Or is she more concerned not to cause unnecessary anxiety to her patients, most of whom will be well at the time they are screened?

And does she have a duty to her patients to **tell them the truth**? Does she have an obligation to tell them what she thinks about the screening programme: does she tell them that she is virtually forced to test by the terms of her contract? Does she tell them beforehand about the uncertainties over false positives (and false negatives)? How much of the truth must she share with her patients (bearing in mind the other potential duty to minimise harm – and that anxiety might be thought to be a harm)?

The blue level

All of the blue boxes deserve scrutiny by GPs. If it turns out that screening produces a true positive result, and if the person is helped by this to avoid a serious disease, then it must be said that the medical procedure has **created autonomy** in that individual. However, if the test is negative, and if it has

---

*Now the Family Health Service Authority (FHSA).

been carried out merely for contractual reasons and the patient has not had this fact properly explained to him, then it is hard to see how medicine has given the patient more control.

If the patient is fully informed of the situation, as the GP herself understands it, and decides anyway to have the test then **autonomy** will have been **respected**. This will be equally so if the patient refuses. However, much hinges upon what the patient understands to be necessary – informed consent can be given only if the patient is truly informed (see Cases 7 and 8).

Screening costs money, and it is not at all clear that it is cost-effective when compared with other scarce treatments available to some on the NHS (for instance, hip replacement operations and kidney dialysis). The GP might have to reassure herself that she is **serving needs first** and, if she decides that she is not, will have to undertake a further, very difficult, ethical analysis about how best to conduct her future practice. Her deliberation might be further complicated by the consideration that by singling out certain groups of people and not all people for screening, she is not **respecting persons equally** but discriminating between her own patients, as well as against those who might benefit from the redirection of funds presently devoted to screening.

This brief discussion of the 'ethics of screening' has deliberately not been presented as a single specific case. There are two reasons for this:

1. It shows that the Ethical Grid can have a general analytical function. Its use need not be restricted only to isolated doctor/patient encounters.

2. At this stage in the book those who have learnt the two basic instruments ought to have gained the confidence to bring real life cases for personal or group analysis.

EXERCISE

You are a GP who regularly screens his patients. A partner, who has read the paper by Mant and Fowler, has come to you with a proposal that the practice ceases to screen patients. Use either the Grid or the Algorithm to help you react to this proposal.

Reference

1. Mant and Fowler (1990) *British Medical Journal*, 300: 916–8.

Case 10

Helping When It's Not Wanted

Introduction

From the early 1960s onwards there has been extensive debate about the nature of mental illness. A variety of positions have been put forward by medical doctors, philosophers, social scientists and historians. By studying the extensive literature[1] on the subject it is possible to detect a wide spectrum of opinion. At one end there are those who believe that mental illness is caused by biochemical abnormalities in the brain, and that some individuals are more genetically susceptible than others,[2] while at the other a school of thought exists that 'mental illness' is a myth, and so psychiatric hospitals are places for detaining social misfits rather than for curing the sick. Convincing evidence either way is very difficult to find.[3] The brain is an enormously complex organism and no-one is able to show how its physical operation produces discrete human thoughts. It is known that some drug therapy can alleviate disturbing mental symptoms, but it does not necessarily follow from this that the symptoms themselves have been caused chemically. Equally, those who consider that there is no such thing as 'mental illness', and that people's mental problems are caused by unfavourable social factors, must explain why some people and not others are adversely affected by similar situations. This group of advocates have also to suggest therapies which are as effective as some drug regimes have been shown to be.

The debate continues. However, what is certain is that millions of people suffer distressing mental symptoms (ranging from mild depression to distressing psychotic phenomena, such as hearing voices or having strong paranoid convictions) for which they need assistance of some kind. When sufferers perceive that they need help, and specifically request it, then ethical problems are not immediately stark. However, as in the case discussed below, sometimes it is not the 'sufferer' who sees a problem, but other people. In such situations doctors have to make a very difficult judgement: should this person be treated against his wishes? Should he be helped even though he says he does not want help?

The Ethics Lecture

Until recently no British medical school offered formal tuition in ethics, although some held informal seminars which could be attended by interested students. Now Britain is beginning to move a little closer to the USA's level of provision of ethics tuition (Departments of Biomedical Ethics are now commonplace in the USA). As ethics teaching develops in this country so medical schools are beginning to employ philosophers, while medical doctors who wish to teach ethics as part of their specialism's clinical attachment are taking advice from Departments of Philosophy.[4] Below is an edited transcript of a talk (including some student responses) on ethics in psychiatry given by a clinician who has learnt to use the Ethical Grid. You should notice that the teacher is being remarkably honest about his feelings and his uncertainties. Such honesty is naturally fostered by genuine use of the Grid.

Dr Loughlin is a senior lecturer in a university Department of Psychiatry. He has secured a three hour session to introduce to the medical students some of the ethical issues which surround the management of psychiatric cases. He is not an expert on ethics but is highly aware of its importance in psychiatry, where issues of involuntary detention and treatment often arise. Although the Mental Health Act 1983 is a powerful guide to appropriate management and tries to protect the rights of patients, it is primarily a legislative rather than an ethical tool. Dr Loughlin feels that there is a danger of using the law as a substitute for ethical analysis. He wishes to demonstrate to the students how to consider the ethical issues surrounding common psychiatric cases and decides to use the Grid as a means by which they can do this. However, he is soon interrupted by one of his students:

'Excuse me, Dr Loughlin, I hope you don't mind, but I think we're a bit confused. Could you say what ethics actually is before you go on? I mean, isn't this a bit of a waste of time actually? Really ethics boils down to a matter of personal opinion, doesn't it?'

Fortunately Dr Loughlin is not thrown by this question. In fact the student's intervention gives him the chance to catch his breath, and to begin again. He explains that it is not easy to find 'objectively right' answers in ethics, but that the important thing is to be as sure as possible that the answer a doctor offers is the best possible in the circumstances. This involves thinking through a range of theories and practical issues in a careful, systematic fashion. And this is what he is going to teach them this afternoon.

He continued, '. . . can I illustrate that point with an example from my own experience? What I have in mind is one of the first cases I ever considered with the aid of the Ethical Grid – the Grid is pictured and explained in your handbooks, don't worry if you've not read about it, I'll explain it fully in a minute. Basically the Grid is a chart to help remind doctors of the extent of issues which we have to consider, and it's also a way of helping us to clarify a situation, choose our priorities, and then justify them if we have to.

'My problem was what to do with Michael, a psychiatric patient I had seen during his two previous hospital admissions, the first of which was about four years ago. Michael was 29 and living at home with his parents. He is an only child and his parents are now in their sixties. They are both retired. The father is an ex-army sergeant, rather short-tempered, and the mother is a meek sort of person who does not enjoy the best of health; she is constantly worrying about her son.

'Michael is schizophrenic, and after his last admission, just under two years ago, was commenced on depot neuroleptic medication basically because of poor compliance with tablets. Up until a few weeks ago Michael had attended the Day Hospital fortnightly for his injection. For some reason, he stopped attending and during this time, as a consequence, was not taking medication. Probably as a result, his behaviour became increasingly bizarre, and unacceptable. He spent long periods alone in his room, often appeared to be talking to himself and occasionally shouted out abuses at passing neighbours. He had also become irritable with his parents and several times had verbally threatened his mother . . . Yes, Maxine isn't it?'

'It sounds to me like he ought to leave home. Can't family circumstances cause psychotic episodes?'

'Some psychiatrists argue that there is evidence that where families are highly critical, hostile and over involved, the risk of relapse in a schizophrenic relative is high.[5] Michael's family, particularly his father, can be a bit like that. For example when Michael stays in bed all day, his father tells him off for being lazy and nags him to do something positive with his life. Such parental attitudes and behaviour can be modified by education, group or family therapy. If this fails, spending time away from home can be protective. Medication in addition to either of these two interventions decreases further the risk of relapse.

'But back to the case. My ethical analysis and intervention were necessary when the Community Psychiatric Nurse was unable to persuade Michael to recommence his medication, nor could she change Michael's mind about returning to hospital. She asked me to make a home visit, which I did. Michael was very agitated, but quite adamant that there was nothing wrong with him. He became very angry, told me to "piss off", and refused any more injections, which he says are uncomfortable and slow him down.

'Michael had obviously deteriorated so, in order to halt his slide, I decided to make a medical recommendation for detention as an involuntary patient under Section 3. To be honest I didn't think too deeply about this decision because I'd known Michael for some years, I knew him to be mentally ill, and I knew that hospital treatment would considerably help him. Funnily enough I had been researching my interest in ethics for some months by then, but I didn't make the connection between my work and ethical analysis straight away, even though my work must involve ethics. It was only when driving back to the hospital that it occurred to me that I ought, for the sake of my conscience, to be able to offer an ethical justification for what I had done.

'Once at home I decided to experiment with the Ethical Grid. I must say I did so with trepidation since it is possible, if you use the Grid as honestly and openly as you can, to discover that you have not adopted the best policy. The Grid can point out to you considerations which had not occurred to you before. As it happened I didn't change my opinion in this case, although I am now slightly less certain than I was at the time that I did the right thing. Er . . . does that worry anybody? . . . Yes?'

'It worries me. If we are going to have to make difficult decision as doctors surely, for our own sakes, we must be totally confident that we've done the right thing. You seem to be saying that it's better to be indecisive . . .'

'Well I can see that it might sound like that, but I'm not. What I am saying is that firm decisions will always have to be made, but also that the decision makers – that is, you in the future – must constantly be able to reflect on those decisions. You must be able to assess them in various ways, and you must be able to be brave enough to say to anybody "I don't know" or even "I was wrong". The important thing is to learn if mistakes have been made, and to try to do better in future.

'In Michael's case my decision might have gone either way. If I had had access to better community resources I might have decided not to recommend a Section but to try something else first. Each case will have some different features – to be flexible and adaptable doesn't mean being inconsistent – so long as one is consistent in trying to think about and justify what one does.

'Let me fill you in on some of the details of my reasoning process over Michael. First the Grid required me to formulate a specific question. That was easy: "should I have Sectioned Michael?" I had a response – Yes – which I then had to test out, in many ways just as if I were checking out a scientific hypothesis. In other words, I could "enter" any of the boxes in order to think the decision through, bearing in mind always that it is up to the user to interpret what each box is to mean in the context.

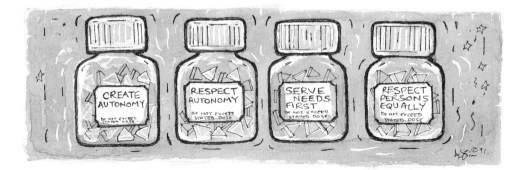

'Then I thought, why not use the Grid as if I was Michael, taking full account of what he had said about himself? I tried this, although I don't think I was able properly to put myself in Michael's shoes. However, after thinking for a while I was drawn into the blue boxes (and this began to worry me, for if Michael were to invoke these boxes – the rationale of health care boxes – then I might be left in a pretty shaky position). Thinking as Michael might have I selected all four blue boxes (which alarmed me!) These are **create autonomy**, **respect autonomy**, **serve needs first**, and **respect persons equally**. I thought that a calm and rational Michael would insist that by treating him against his wishes I was obviously not **respecting autonomy**, by removing his liberty I was obviously not **creating autonomy**, by taking him away from his home I was not meeting his basic **need**, and that by singling him out and by siding with his parents I was obviously not **respecting persons equally**. It seemed to me that Michael could also claim that I was not **minimising harm** either; from his point of view, the injection was an uncomfortable procedure, and made him feel slowed down.

'But then it occurred to me that all this missed the point, and that I too could use blue boxes to justify my actual policy. The point is that at the time Michael was not calm and rational, far from it, and that the whole point of my intervention was to try to ensure that Michael again became calm and rational as quickly as possible. In other words, I decided not to respect Michael's autonomy because I did not think he was in a position to make rational, informed choices. My aim was to restore him to a mental state where this was possible again, that is to **create autonomy**. There were other considerations too. Michael's parents were under a great deal of stress. His mother was a frail lady and Michael had been verbally threatening to her already. There was a real danger that during such an incident, his father may have lost his temper and physically assaulted Michael. I could not see how such a scenario – which had occurred during a previous relapse – would **benefit** Michael or his parents. Moreover, his behaviour was reducing the threshold of tolerance of the neighbours and hardly helped the image of mental illness or psychiatrists for that matter! So, I concluded that letting him stay at home in his present state would certainly not result in a **beneficial outcome** for Michael, his family, his neighbours and indeed psychiatry. I also considered **the risk**. I wanted not only to detain Michael but also compulsorily treat him with neuroleptic drugs which are known to have short term and long term side-effects. But I considered that I could justify those side-effects because I was carrying out my duty to **minimise harm**, both by helping Michael to get better and careful monitoring of his response to medications.'

'Did you tell Michael about the side-effects of the medication?'

'Michael was already aware of the side-effects since he had been on these drugs for some years. However, you do raise a thorny issue here which is how much you tell a patient about side-effects when you know they do not want the medication anyway. What do people here think one should do about that? Yes, Maxine . . .'

'I think patients whether they are psychiatrically ill or not have a right to know about all the possible effects of medication they receive.'

'But if you tell them,' another student chipped in, 'they might refuse to take medication which they need. However, you could give them all the information once they are better.'

Dr Loughlin: 'So you seem to be saying, Bill, that when the capacity for making rational decisions has been restored, you can give back the choice to the patient. Can anyone see anything wrong with that approach?'

'Well, you could be sued at a later date for not telling patients all the side-effects when they first receive them.'

'Yes, that's certainly happened in the USA and if litigation continues to increase in this country, it might occur here in the future.'

'But don't you think . . .'

EXERCISE

1. Make out a case for telling Michael all the side-effects of the neuroleptics he is going to receive in hospital, using the Grid.

2. Use the Grid to justify not telling him.

EXERCISE

Donald has exactly the same problems as Michael, and is in exactly the same situation – but with one difference: his parents are very supportive of him, despite his attacks on them, and will do anything not to have their son enter a mental hospital.

1. Use the Grid to argue the parent's case against Sectioning.

2. Use the Grid to justify (if possible) Sectioning Donald despite his parents' protests.

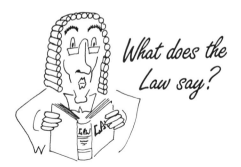

What does the Law say?

Mental Health Act 1983, Section 3, Admission for Treatment

Detention under this Act can last six months and may be extended following review. An application by the nearest relative or an approved social worker is required. Two medical recommendations are also required, one from an approved doctor (that is, usually a psychiatrist with a higher qualification). The other doctor should generally be the patient's family doctor. The grounds for detention are:

(a)   The patient is suffering from a mental illness, severe mental impairment, psychopathic disorder or mental impairment that makes it appropriate to receive treatment in hospital; and

continued

continued

(b) in the case of psychopathic disorder or mental impairment, such treatment is likely to alleviate or prevent deterioration of his condition; and

(c) it is necessary for the health and safety of the patient or for the protection of other persons that he should receive such treatment, and it cannot be provided unless he is detained under a Section.

References

1. Beauchamp, T.L. and Childress, J.F. (1983) *Principles of Biomedical Ethics*. Oxford: Oxford University Press.
2. Bloch, S. and Chidoff, P. (1981) *Psychiatric Ethics*. Oxford: Oxford University Press.
3. Edwards, R.B. (1982) *Psychiatry and Ethics*. Buffalo: Prometheus Books.
4. Seedhouse, D.F. (1988) *Ethics: The Heart of Health Care*. Chichester: John Wiley and Sons.
5. Vaughn, C.E. and Leff J.P. (1976) The influence of family and social factors on the course of psychiatric illness: a comparison of schizophrenic and depressed neurotic patients. *British Journal of Psychiatry* 129: 125–37.

Case 11

A Consultation with an 'Ethicist'

This case describes the correspondence between a consultant psychiatrist and a philosopher who specialises in health care ethics. The consultant is employed by a Special Hospital and has become worried about the treatment of a sex offender in his Unit. He has particular doubts about the scientific and ethical validity of one part of the treatment programme, which is being used as a type of test. He has written to the philosopher describing the case and· requesting an ethical analysis.

The philosopher's response is given below. The Ethical Grid was employed to assist the moral reasoning process. Naturally the philosopher gave a considered, but personal, judgement. His is not necessarily the best opinion (more technically, it does not necessarily *create the highest degree of morality*). Readers who disagree with it might wish to challenge the philosopher's deliberation either through use of the Grid or the Algorithm, or according to an alternative methodology if preferred.

This case offers the most developed and sustained ethical analysis in this casebook, but even so some professional philosophers would find it quite unsophisticated. It might be said that such a response would confuse simple style with simple argument. However, those readers who wish to study technical analyses in medical ethics should turn to the professional journals.

The Case of Nigel Brown

21 January 1992

Park Side Hospital
Park Ridge
Manchester
MA37 3NW

DPH/HAS

Dear Dr Home,

re: Nigel Brown

I wonder if I might ask your opinion about the case of a patient under my charge? I am concerned that what is happening to him is unethical.

I am a consultant psychiatrist at the above Special Hospital. As you may know there are four other Special Hospitals in England (Broadmoor, Rampton, Park Lane and Moss Side) funded directly by the Department of Health, providing facilities for the treatment and confinement of dangerous psychiatric patients. Patients with a wide range of diagnoses (including psychotic, psychopathic, and mentally handicapped people) are involuntarily detained in these institutions. Some are admitted because they have posed severe management problems for other establishments; however, a large proportion have committed serious offences including homicide, serious physical assault on others, arson, and rape. A considerable number of the patients have sexually offended against young children, sometimes repeatedly and with violence. Nigel Brown is a fairly typical sex offender. On more than one occasion he has been arrested for sexually abusing young boys and he has served several jail sentences as a consequence. Although not particularly bright he had been able to look after himself and had held down a series of jobs between these periods of incarceration. He was not violent towards the boys he molested but rather resorted to bribery in order to persuade them to co-operate. His victims ranged from between nine and thirteen years of age. Like many sex offenders, Nigel was polite and courteous in his manner and posed no serious problems for the hospital staff. He had been admitted (by my predecessor) to the hospital three days before his last sentence had been due to expire, and when first seen by the psychologist and myself had been in the hospital for approximately two years.

The provision of worthwhile therapy is a constant problem within Special Hospitals. Because of limited resources much of the work takes the form of assessments designed to determine

continued

continued

whether the patient remains dangerous to others. One assessment used with sex offenders is the penis plethysmograph. Briefly, this involves exposing the patient to sexually arousing (pornographic) material and monitoring his response by means of a strain gauge placed around his penis. This technique is far from fail-safe but, by the use of appropriate material (including child pornography), it can provide useful information about the patient's sexual interests. Data obtained by this method may be presented to a Mental Health Review Tribunal when it sits to consider whether a patient should be released from the hospital. Nigel was offered such an assessment prior to the tribunal. However, the choice of whether or not to co-operate was clearly a difficult one for him. Nigel explained that he had 'paid his debt to society' and deeply resented serving an extra two years in addition to his prison term. Moreover, he knew that if he agreed to the assessment and showed evidence of a continuing sexual interest in children his already slim chances of release would be diminished further. On the other hand, it was doubtful whether the tribunal would agree to release him knowing that he had refused to take part. Nigel was thus exposed to a kind of double-jeopardy.

In fact Nigel refused the assessment. Despite Nigel's good conduct in the hospital, and despite no clear clinical evidence of mental disorder, the tribunal declined to recommend his release. Other patients facing the same dilemma have often expressed the opinion that they have no choice but to co-operate.

I should add that the Tribunal fudged the issue of which mental disorder Nigel is suffering from. I have found that this happens from time to time, and all that is then clear is that in the Tribunal's view the patient continues to be 'mentally ill'.

You should also know that I have spoken with Nigel on several occasions. He consistently denies any sexual interest in boys, but in my view (which is based on 25 years' experience) this interest remains despite 'masturbatory reconditioning' and other therapy, and I think that it will be with Nigel for life. Presumably this is why he decided to refuse the test.

Could you provide me with an analysis of the ethics of this practice? It could prove influential since the Hospital is to review this, and other assessment procedures, in April. If you require any further information please contact me by 'phone. I shall, of course, be happy to pay your usual fee.

Yours sincerely,

P. Harper

Daniel Harper, MRCPsych

9 February 1992
Department of Philosophy
University of Casterbridge
Casterbridge
CA4 9JG

DFH/EMF

Dear Dr Harper,

re: <u>The Case of Nigel Brown</u>

Thank you for your recent request for an ethical analysis. I
have thought the case through using a method recommended by a
colleague, Dr Seedhouse. You will, I'm sure, bear in mind that
although I am satisfied that this analysis can withstand any
challenge that I can think of, it is not necessarily the *right*
answer. Other philosophers might present other arguments (just
as is the case with clinical discussion, I believe) but I feel
that there would be a clear majority verdict amongst ethicists
over my assessment of this case (although I might add that most
would not be as thorough as I!).

First of all it is important to clarify the *key aspects* of the
case. These seem to be:

(i)   Nigel's involuntary confinement in hospital (he has served
        a prison sentence after which he was not released but was
        confined under Section Three of the Mental Health Act
        1983);
(ii)   The nature of his offence (why is this somehow a 'special'
        offence?);
(iii)   The treatment offered by the hospital (what 'curative'
        treatment was given? What rehabilitative help? Was the
        role of the health workers in fact only or primarily to
        assess?);
(iv)   The plethysmographic assessment (how is this relevant?
        What is being assessed?);
(v)   The 'double-jeopardy' issue; and
(vi)   The validity of the authority of the Mental Health Review
        Tribunal over Nigel Brown.

Naturally the selection of these key aspects reflects my
prejudices. However, the selection of some key aspect is a
necessary starting point of any analysis. Each can be assessed
and challenged by a proper use of the Ethical Grid, and it may
be that, after deliberation, they are no longer considered to
be central. Other analysts might have highlighted the issue
of child abuse, and might therefore have chosen to focus

continued

continued

primarily upon the risks that Nigel Brown could pose to children if released. However, whatever the starting point, any analyst who uses the Grid must pay attention to the four coloured layers, and in the process must examine the strength of his position in relation to alternatives. It must be remembered that a condition of use of the Grid is that it must be applied honestly in the hope of reaching a decision which will enhance the potentials of as many people as is practically possible.

Before one is able to use the Grid it is essential to arrive at a clear decision about *the best question to ask*. The Grid *must* have a clear focus. This is because examples such as Nigel's present a whole web of moral dilemmas (What should a psychiatrist do? How should the Tribunal deliberate? What should Nigel do?). In this case I have chosen to ask: *should the Tribunal have recommended Nigel's release despite his refusal to undergo the plethysmographic assessment?* I believe that by answering this specific question I will, at the same time, be able to address your general concern about the ethics of the procedure.

The choice that faced the members of the Tribunal was stark: to let Nigel Brown go or to keep him locked up for an indefinite period. If Nigel is released he might take his chances in life as a free man and never again break the law. Alternatively he might revert to his previous behaviour or even find more violent ways of assaulting children. If he remains in detention he will have fewer civil rights than a criminal, apparently he will continue to be stigmatised and institutionalised, and his opportunities for fulfilment will be severely limited.

My core analysis

I first considered the black layer of the Grid, which deals with external considerations, and homed in on the box **the degree of certainty of the evidence on which action is taken**. Presumably there were other tests but it appears from what you say that Nigel's refusal to submit to the penis plethysmograph was crucial to the issue of his release. But what is this refusal evidence of? It might have been that Nigel found the thought of the test unpleasant in itself, but it is more likely that he believed that he would 'fail' it – that is, he believed that he would be sexually aroused by child pornography – and that this would mean that he would not be set free. And if the had taken the test and failed it, what would this have been evidence of? The only legitimate conclusion that might be drawn from this outcome would have been that Nigel Brown is sexually excited by child sexual stimuli, and perhaps by other sexual stimuli as well. The Tribunal must already have been aware that this result was highly likely, but this virtual certainty cannot be taken to generate a further certainty that Nigel will act on his impulses. Unless treatment to control his sexual drive has been successful (and

continued

continued

your strong suspicion is that it has not), nothing could be less surprising than Nigel becoming excited by the pornographic stimuli.

It seems to me that Nigel's sexual inclinations should not have been the issue. A more appropriate topic for review would have been whether or not Nigel was *likely to act on his impulses* or whether he was more in control of his behaviour, or at least more afraid of the consequences of offending. In short, I consider the evidence of the assessment irrelevant to Nigel's release unless it could show beyond reasonable doubt that he is mentally disordered, or that molestation is likely to re-occur.

There is a further cause for concern about the test, which should give you some pause for thought. The test is used to assess whether or not a particular person has undesirable sexual inclinations. If he is found to have such inclinations then this discovery can have serious implications for his liberty. But this policy has an obvious logical extension. What would the Tribunal have decided if Nigel no longer responded to the child pornography, but was found to be aroused by acts of sadism or bestiality? This arousal might have been taken to be an indication that Nigel had become a danger to others for a new reason, and it does not seem unreasonable to assume that this evidence might then be considered a ground for his continued detention. However, if this is the case then there seems no reason, other than scarcity of resources, to restrict the test to sex offenders. If the general public is to be properly protected then perhaps this sort of test should be applied to all prison inmates when their release is up for consideration.

I next thought over the box labelled **the law** to see if further progress could be made. Since it is known that the Tribunal did not recommend Nigel's release it must be assumed that it considered that he was 'suffering from a mental disorder of a nature or degree which warranted detention in hospital for either assessment or treatment, and that he should be detained in the interests of his own health and safety or with a view to the protection of others' as required by the Mental Health Act (Section 3).

Nigel was convicted for bribing boys for sex, a form of behaviour which is illegal in Great Britain. He served a prison sentence. Three days before his release he was Sectioned to a Special Hospital — so, instantly it seems, he was no longer regarded as a criminal but as mentally disordered. His status changed and he lost the civil liberties accorded to people, including criminals, who are not said to be mentally disordered. So what happened? Did he sexually abuse any more boys? There was no opportunity for this in prison. Did he have a psychotic or neurotic episode, or some change in his personality? I understand from our recent 'phone conversation that the evidence here is ambiguous, and in some dispute.

continued

continued

What seems to have happened is that 'the authorities' (presumably the prison social worker and two medical practitioners) applied to have Nigel Brown detained on the ground that he was mentally disordered and a danger to others. What seems to have happened, in other words, is that Nigel was assessed as having a mental disorder (and so as not being responsible for his actions) on the grounds of the very same behaviour that the courts previously had regarded as illegal (and so held him responsible for). Of course I may be being quite naive on this, but there is at least a probability that in the end Nigel was not even to be judged on his actions, but on his refusal to take a test which, if he did take and fail it, could only add more credibility to the existing belief that he has a sexual appetite for boys. If things remain the same it is hard to see how he will ever be released.

What are the broader implications of this bizarre illogic? The penal system is said to exist to punish, but also to rehabilitate people so that afterwards they can go on to do other things in their lives. It is crucial to this system that once a person has been punished then he must be set free. He may offend again but this is a risk that any non-totalitarian society must take. If the punishment has been a positive experience, and thoughtful rehabilitation has been attempted, it is to be hoped that there will be less risk that the person will commit a similar offence.

Why, then, does there seem to be one rule for sex offenders and another for all other categories of criminal? Should a person who has committed armed robbery on three banks and has been gaoled for each offence be kept in gaol until society can be sure that he will no longer rob banks? Bank robbers are not, as a rule, shown videos of bank robberies to see if they are excessively interested by them (sexually or otherwise) before they are released from custody. Why are sex offenders a special case? Is sexual molestation somehow more inherently wrong, or are the consequences of such activity so much more awful than serious non-sexual assaults on children?

Still in the black layer I tried to assess **the risk**. The correct question to ask here is, 'what risk and to whom?'. If Nigel were to be released it must be accepted that there is a substantial risk that he would again attempt to abuse young boys sexually. But there are other risks to be considered. There is a risk that Nigel will become incarcerated for life, and that he will become so demoralised, and so indelibly labelled as a 'sex offender', that he will never be rehabilitated even if eventually set free. And there is also a risk to the Tribunal and to the authority that it represents. If Nigel is released and lives a normal life hardly anyone will notice, but if he is allowed his liberty and commits further offences there might well be unfavourable publicity. Such publicity might undermine the future ability of the Tribunal to perform its task.

This brief summary of risks drew my attention to the green layer of the Ethical Grid, which is concerned with *consequences*: there seems to be a disharmony between the boxes **most beneficial**

continued

continued

outcome for the patient, most beneficial outcome for society and most beneficial outcome for a particular group. The individual in question is Nigel and the group is the set of boys between the ages of nine and thirteen who are potentially at risk. It may be that the Tribunal feels obliged to protect society at large by continuing to restrain Nigel but, specifically, the main conflict of interest must lie between Nigel and the boys. You will remember that the task of health workers (and it must be the case, by definition, that a Mental Health Review Tribunal falls into this category) is to remove or prevent obstacles which stand in the way of individuals achieving their potential (see below[1]). However, although the Tribunal appears to have emphasised consequences in its deliberations the green level of the Grid is not a particularly fruitful source of analysis since no benefits are being increased – the only consequences appear to be bad ones – there is no *positive* emphasis. And further it is not clear how severe each bad consequence might be. Not only is the effect of continued confinement for Nigel unknown, but also it is unclear (to me at least) what bad effects the sexual molestations may have caused to boys in the past, or might cause other boys in the future.

It seems more accurate to assume that the Tribunal has worked on the principle that it has a duty to **minimise harm** (in the red layer of the Grid). I agree that this is the appropriate duty in this case but, the nature of the harm to be minimised is unclear and needs to be questioned. Presumably the Tribunal decided to minimise harm to boys – to take the safety first option – by extending Nigel's 'sentence', judging that the potential harm to boys outweighed the actual harm to Nigel's liberty, happiness and opportunity for development.

But does this opinion create *the highest degree of morality*? The Tribunal is not a court of law but a proper part of a Mental Health Service, and so bound by the rationale of work for health. Thus it is vital to move into the blue layer. I chose to begin with the box **create autonomy**.

Given your information about the lack of resources for care in Special Hospitals – that many patients in the hospitals are there merely because of management problems, and that sexual offenders are not as a rule treated with a view to rehabilitation but assessed to see if they are no longer dangerous – I conclude that very little – or at least not enough – has been done to enable Nigel to take more control over his life.

Appropriate care would include positive courses of broad education, the enhancement of Nigel's practical skills, the provision of the means by which Nigel might develop new interests (which might give him better employment prospects, and open possibilities for different social networks), and the where-withal for him to see himself as part of a community.

Unless more resources are made available it is unlikely that Nigel's autonomy can be improved within the hospital, although it could be improved at a stroke by his release. It may be that life will be hard outside the institution for someone with his record but his freedoms – for example, the freedom to associate,

continued

continued

to seek work, to travel and to explore other possibilities – might be immeasurably improved. What is more this is what Nigel Brown wants. He knows the implications of release and he prefers it. It should fall to the Tribunal to **respect autonomy** – to respect Nigel's wishes – unless they can justify why they should not.

Conclusion and recommendation

I have followed through a process of moral reasoning using the Ethical Grid based on information supplied by you. Perhaps this case has not been particularly representative of the use of the Grid because my initial views were progressively hardened by the analysis. This does not necessarily happen during moral reasoning. Indeed, flexibility and change is normally encouraged in the process. It is almost as common for a person who uses the Ethical Grid properly to change her mind as it is for her to gain a more articulate means to justify her original position.

However, you have come to me for an opinion – not a philosophy seminar. In answer to the question 'should the Tribunal have recommended Nigel's release in the light of his refusal to undergo the assessment?' I have selected the following boxes from the Ethical Grid as the most salient: **the law**, **the degree of certainty of the evidence on which action is taken**, **create autonomy**, and **respect autonomy**. In sum, I believe that Nigel is being restrained without justification (and incidentally in abuse of Mental Health legislation since he committed a criminal offence which is not regarded as indicative of a mental disorder, and there is no firm evidence of a mental disorder occurring during his spell of imprisonment). The evidence on which he is now held is primarily his refusal to take a test which may not be a valid indicator of his future behaviour (you will be better placed to judge this than I), and which can provide little new information about his sexual inclinations. Nigel is not being empowered to take better control of his life; rather he continues to be emasculated by his incarceration. Above all else he wants to be free and this is being denied him, not genuinely on the ground that he is ill but on the ground that there is a chance that if he were to be released he would again commit the criminal offence of bribing boys for sex. If it is right that Nigel should be held because he might commit a criminal offence in future then, it might be argued, it must surely be right that any one of the rest of us should be so restrained. Yes. Nigel Brown should have been released. This would have produced a higher degree of morality.

In answer to your general question – the use of the plethysmo-graph is ethically dubious. A better method ought to be found.

Yours sincerely.

D. Horne.

Dr Home, BA, PhD

EXERCISE

1. Whether you agree with Dr Home or not, attempt to produce an
    ethical analysis which addresses the question: should Nigel Brown
    be detained in hospital until he poses the same level of risk to
    children as the 'man in the street' (i.e. until Nigel can be clearly said
    to be normal).

2. It may be that you have more information about Special Hospitals
    available to you than Dr Home did. If so, point out flaws in Dr Home's
    analysis and incorporate your objections into a Grid-based argument
    of your own addressing Home's specifically expressed question.

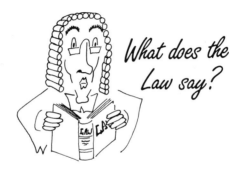

**Mental Health Act 1983, Section 47, removal to hospital of persons
serving sentence of imprisonment etc.**

Application:

By reports from at least two medical practitioners to the Secretary of
State:

   The Home Secretary may make a 'transfer direction' that a person
serving a sentence of imprisonment shall be removed to, and detained
in, such a hospital (not being a mental nursing home) as he may specify
in the direction, provided that he is satisfied (by reports from two doctors,
one of whom is approved) that:

(a)   The person named is suffering from one of the four forms of mental
      disorder.
(b)   The disorder is of a nature or degree which makes hospital treatment
      under detention appropriate.

continued

continued

(c) In the case of psychopathic disorder or mental impairment, that treatment is likely to alleviate or prevent deterioration of the condition.

(d) That, having regard to the public interest and all circumstances, a 'transfer direction' is expedient.

Special notes:

(a) A restriction direction on the person's discharge may be made by the Home Secretary (Section 49) (similar to a restriction order).

(b) The person must be transferred within 14 days, or the transfer direction lapses.

(c) There is a right of appeal to the Mental Health Review Tribunal within the first six months and during each subsequent period of detention (this applies to persons either with or without restriction directions).

Duration:

The Home Secretary may order the person to be returned to prison if he is informed that the person has recovered or that no further effective treatment can be given.

This information/advice may be conveyed to him from:

(a) The regional medical officer
(b) Any other registered medical practitioner
(c) A Mental Health Review Tribunal

Reference

1. Seedhouse, D.F. (1986) *Health: The Foundations for Achievement.* Chichester: John Wiley and Sons.

Case 12

Abortion

Abortion is perhaps the most emotive issue of all in medical ethics. People tend to have well-formed and strongly held opinions, and it is rare to find individuals flexible enough about the topic to be open to persuasion. It is far more common, unfortunately, for discussion about the pros and cons of abortion to degenerate into arguments where people come to be at loggerheads with each other – often fiercely so. In such circumstances people assert rigid stances and usually, sooner or later, each side accuses the other of being utterly immoral: stalemate!

As in most theoretical debate about ethical issues a spectrum, with extremes, can be identified. In the case of abortion the poles consist of unshakeably pro- or anti-abortion supporters. It is a reasonably accurate generalisation to say that those in favour of abortion tend to base their case on what they describe as 'the fundamental right of a women to do as she chooses with her own body', while those opposed to abortion stress 'the right to life of the fetus' (sometimes the anti-abortion lobby tries to make political capital by raising a semantic issue, calling the 'fetus' a 'baby' or a 'child', often even from the moment of conception).

When members of the two extreme groups talk about abortion it is simply *inevitable* that they will not agree. For however long they converse with (or shout at) each other they will not move closer. Why should this be?

The reason for the deadlock is quite simple: there is no *empirical* way to decide which group is 'right'. The dispute is irresolvable because theoretical moral questions of this sort cannot be decided by appeal to factual evidence. Basically two major theoretical questions are at issue. These are:

> 1. Do women actually have a moral right to dispose of potential people?
>
> 2. What is the 'moral status' of the fetus? (If the fetus is a 'person' rather than a cluster of insentient cells then the implications for the way it is treated will be different – but there is no laboratory test available to answer this question.)

In order to tackle such philosophical puzzles it is necessary to embark on high level, technical theoretical analysis of a kind not even touched on in this casebook. However, even though these questions are extremely complicated and difficult to answer, this does not mean that doctors are unable to carry out ethical analysis in specific situations. On the contrary, each potential abortion case is unique, and there are always a range of considerations – both practical and theoretical – to reflect upon before reaching a decision. Although not every issue can be resolved with certainty, it is, nevertheless, possible for a doctor to reach an intelligent decision which he can justify.

Joanna

Joanna's case does not rest solely on the theoretical rights and wrongs of the abortion debate. Certainly it is necessary and important to consider the status of the fetus in any deliberation about how to act for the best, but this is not the only consideration – neither is it always the *central* consideration of the doctor's ethical analysis.

Joanna Curtis is a 15 year old school girl. She is very bright, has great sporting ability, and is attractive and mature for her age. She has been going out with Jack for a little over a year. They are obviously in love in the peculiarly intense way that teenagers can be. The relationship has increasingly worried Joanna's parents, who have encouraged Joanna to call it off. But the more they have tried to dissuade her the more obsessed and consumed their daughter has seemed to become.

Mr and Mrs Curtis recently went to visit Jack's parents, John and Wendy Johnson, but this did their cause more harm than good. Clive and Celia Curtis are both wealthy, public school educated people who own a large and successful retail business, while the Johnsons are solidly 'working class'. John is a factory worker, and both husband and wife are active members of the Labour Party.

The Curtis's explained, they thought as tactfully as they could, their great concern for Joanna's future. They spoke about their daughter's exceptional talents, and talked of the fantastic opportunities she could expect in life if she continued her studies and went to university. Their fear, they said, is that Joanna will leave school and set up home with or even marry Jack, and that this will be a disaster for both children in the long run. The Johnsons reacted angrily to this implicit criticism of Jack: neither are children, Jack will be 18 in a few months, what they choose to do is their business – and all the best to them.

Joanna is furious when her parents tell her about the visit on their return. A row develops, until she virtually spits the fact at her parents that she is pregnant. Horrified, Mr and Mrs Curtis say that there will be no recriminations, that she must go to Dr Williams tomorrow – she'll confirm it and make the arrangements.

'What arrangements?'

'For the termination of course.'

'Oh no, I'm not having an abortion, I'm having our baby.'

After much persuasion and pressure Joanna agrees to accompany her mother and father to Dr Williams' surgery. A pregnancy test is performed and proves positive. The family put forward their conflicting points of view, and Dr Williams quickly sees the need for diplomacy. She makes neutral noises to both sides, and confesses that she needs time to think very carefully about what she might do to help them.

Dr Williams decides to turn to the Algorithm for assistance. She turns first to the External Considerations. Clearly Joanna is pregnant, and Dr Williams is now well aware of the wishes of her parents. However, she knows nothing directly of the wishes of the father. Perhaps he ought to be considered?

Dr Williams is very familiar with the Abortion Act and its inherent ambiguity (see What does the Law Say? below). She knows of one local obstetrician who performs abortions 'on demand', and she knows too that by simply writing down 'pregnancy' as the medical ground for the justification of an operation she is very unlikely to be successfully prosecuted by the 'pro-life' movement. The onus would be on the instigators of any prosecution to prove false the currently accepted medical wisdom – that abortion within 12 weeks is safer than childbirth.[1,2] They would also need to demonstrate that Dr Williams had acted in bad faith, for instance, by showing that she did not believe the statistics, but went ahead anyway.

But, she thinks, this is all besides the point. To perform an abortion on an obviously unwilling 15 year old would surely constitute a serious criminal assault. But presumably this is not the sort of assistance which Mr and Mrs Curtis require. In Dr Williams' view the Curtis's want her help to pressurise Joanna – to coerce her into having an abortion. This places her in a difficult position, but not one where she must deliberate about abortion *per se*, but one where she must decide whether to help force Joanna to act in opposition to her present wishes. Dr Williams takes the same long-term outlook as Joanna's parents, but should she try to impose her point of view on the girl?

Now that she is more clear about her focus – about the question she is addressing, Dr Williams continues to move within the Algorithm. Having made little progress within the External Considerations segment she moves into Moral Duties. She thinks about **doing positive good** and **minimising harm**, which seem to be the most relevant duties. Of course, it is up to the doctor to define both 'good' and 'harm'. Is having a baby a 'harm'? Is it a 'good'? Is abortion a 'harm'? Is there a distinction to be made between long-term and short-term good or harm? Dr Williams has identified many major questions, but needs to simplify the problem. It is just too big for her to handle. Perhaps the clarification of outcomes is the best next step? She turns to Consequences.

What is the priority here? Certainly it is not herself, and Dr Williams does not think that the single case of Joanna has major social ramifications. It is between the four of them, and the onus is on Dr Williams. Should she be neutral, should she side with the parents (with whom she agrees), or should she side with Joanna against her mother and father (she is out-numbered and out-gunned at the moment). What is the priority then? Is it the group (either the family, or the family and the doctor) or is it the patient (or potential patient) – Joanna? Dr Williams can understand a case for her treating the family as a group and recommending that they all receive counselling help to make a collective decision. But, she considers against this that they do not have a medical problem, they have a family problem, and she does not feel her position as a clinician entitles her to intervene to this extent. Joanna must be the priority then? So the answer must be that she should respect Joanna's autonomy, which would also be a legally safe option.

Knowing that considerations of autonomy feature in the Central Conditions of Health Work, Dr Williams shifts her gaze to this segment, but then stops abruptly. No. That's not right. Joanna isn't the priority either. No-one is the priority! If she is not legitimised as a clinician to intervene in the family problem because it is not medical (although it would require a medical intervention to carry out the abortion), then neither is she sanctioned to advocate for Joanna. Pregnancy is not a disease and it is to disease that doctors primarily attend.

Dr Williams moves out of the Algorithm, not to the Final Common Pathway, but just out of it. She realises that she was deliberating about a problem where she had no role, and she thinks that she has learnt an important lesson.

EXERCISE

Although Dr Williams has taken this decision many doctors would understandably feel obliged to help. You are a doctor of this type. Continue with your journey through the Algorithm. Explore the Central Conditions of Health Work, and then continue to circle until you feel able to join the Final Common Pathway.

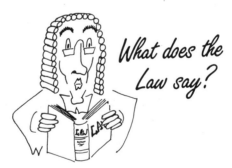

What does the Law say?

The Abortion Act 1967

Medical termination of pregnancy

Section 1:

(1)   Subject to the provisions of this section, a person shall not be guilty of an offence under the law relating to abortion when a pregnancy is terminated by a registered medical practitioner if two registered medical practitioners are of the opinion, formed in good faith –

continued

continued

(a) that the continuance of the pregnancy would involve risk to the life of the pregnant woman, or of injury to the physical or mental health of the pregnant woman or any existing children of her family, greater than if the pregnancy were terminated; or

(b) that there is substantial risk that if the child were born it would suffer from such physical or mental abnormalities as to be seriously handicapped.

(2) In determining whether the continuance of a pregnancy would involve such risk of injury to health as is mentioned in paragraph (a) of subsection (1) of this section, account may be taken of the pregnant woman's actual or reasonably foreseeable environment.

(3) Except as provided by subsection (4) of this section, any treatment for the termination of pregnancy must be carried out in a hospital vested in [the Secretary of State for the purposes of his functions under the National Health Services Act 1977 or the National Health Service (Scotland) Act 1978 or in a place approved for the purposes of this section by the Secretary of State].

(4) Subsection (3) of this section, and so much of subsection (1) as relates to the opinion of two registered medical practitioners, shall not apply to the termination of a pregnancy by a registered medical practitioner in a case where he is of the opinion, formed in good faith, that the termination is immediately necessary to save the life or to prevent grave permanent injury to the physical or mental health of the pregnant woman.

Conscientious objection to participation in treatment

Section 4:

(1) Subject to subsection (2) of this section, no person shall be under any duty, whether by contract or by any statutory or other legal requirement, to participate in any treatment authorised by this Act to which he has a conscientious objection:
Provided that in legal proceedings the burden of proof of conscientious objection shall rest on the person claiming to rely in it.

(2) Nothing in subsection (1) of this section shall affect any duty to participate in treatment which is necessary to save the life or to prevent grave permanent injury to the physical or mental health of a pregnant woman.

(3) In any proceedings before a court in Scotland, a statement on oath by any person to the effect that he has a conscientious objection to participating in any treatment authorised by this Act shall be sufficient evidence for the purpose of discharging the burden of proof imposed upon him by subsection (1) of this section.

continued on next page

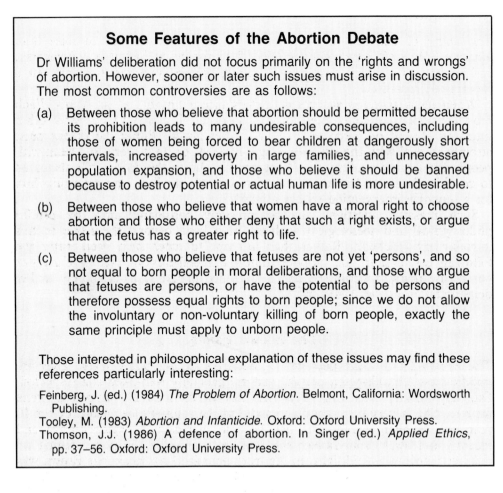

continued

The Law in Relation to Under-16s

At present the law is this: the doctor should 'make every effort to involve the parents', but if a girl is intelligent and mature enough to understand what is involved in the operation, the doctor, if the girl insists on not telling her parents or if they refuse to agree to an abortion, may go ahead on the basis of the girl's consent alone.

Some Features of the Abortion Debate

Dr Williams' deliberation did not focus primarily on the 'rights and wrongs' of abortion. However, sooner or later such issues must arise in discussion. The most common controversies are as follows:

(a) Between those who believe that abortion should be permitted because its prohibition leads to many undesirable consequences, including those of women being forced to bear children at dangerously short intervals, increased poverty in large families, and unnecessary population expansion, and those who believe it should be banned because to destroy potential or actual human life is more undesirable.

(b) Between those who believe that women have a moral right to choose abortion and those who either deny that such a right exists, or argue that the fetus has a greater right to life.

(c) Between those who believe that fetuses are not yet 'persons', and so not equal to born people in moral deliberations, and those who argue that fetuses are persons, or have the potential to be persons and therefore possess equal rights to born people; since we do not allow the involuntary or non-voluntary killing of born people, exactly the same principle must apply to unborn people.

Those interested in philosophical explanation of these issues may find these references particularly interesting:

Feinberg, J. (ed.) (1984) *The Problem of Abortion.* Belmont, California: Wordsworth Publishing.
Tooley, M. (1983) *Abortion and Infanticide.* Oxford: Oxford University Press.
Thomson, J.J. (1986) A defence of abortion. In Singer (ed.) *Applied Ethics,* pp. 37–56. Oxford: Oxford University Press.

References

1. R. v Smith (John) (1974) 1.W.L.R. 1510CA.
2. Munday, D., Francome, C. and Savage, W. (1989) Twenty-one years of legal abortion. *British Medical Journal* 298: 1231–4.

Case 13

Child Abuse

Introduction

The abuse of children, sexually or otherwise, is guaranteed to raise high emotion.[1] More often than not doctors find themselves at the hub of controversy, and in any case where suspicion is strong will be required to carry out a medical examination.

When child abuse is suspected doctors face a number of problems. Each must consider what constitutes abuse, who to tell (if anybody), and what other measures should be taken to prevent further abuse. Either the doctor must attempt to deal with the situation single-handed, or must work in a team with people from other professions. Whatever his choice the doctor will also need to consider limits to his role – how far does his medical training equip him for a sensitive intervention within a family?

Such massive questions can be properly considered only by careful philosophical and sociological analysis, of a kind beyond the scope of this introductory casebook. Rather than attempt to enter such deep water the following case is short and simply outlined. It represents one pattern of analysis out of the many possibilities, and is intended primarily to offer one further demonstration of the Algorithm.

The Brown Family

The Brown family have been on Dr Munro's list for many years. They are middle-class, church-going people, and are generally well-liked and respected. One day shortly after Christmas Mrs Brown consults Dr Munro in some distress. She is very concerned about the uncharacteristic behaviour of her 10 year old daugher Annie. She has become increasingly argumentative and recently ran away from home: she was discovered by the police sitting on children's swings at midnight, in the freezing cold. Last week Mrs Brown was asked to go to Annie's school, where the headmaster informed her that Annie had been showing signs of marked sexualised behaviour, reflected in her play, and she had begun to reveal precocious sexual knowledge in her talk both to other children and to teachers. It was the headmaster who had suggested that Mrs Brown ought to speak to her GP about Annie.

Dr Munro's suspicion is that Annie has been the victim of sexual abuse. What action should he take? What ethical issues should he consider?

Dr Munro recognises that he is no expert in the diagnosis and investigation of child sexual abuse (CSA). However, so great are the potential ramifications in this sort of case that he feels that it is essential to assemble as many facts as possible before taking any action. After he has elicited a comprehensive history from the mother he asks to see Annie, accompanied by Mrs Brown, the next day. This interview reveals little further relevant information but he continues to have some cause to suspect that CSA has occurred. Dr Munro still wishes for more information, and so asks Mrs Brown for permission to contact Annie's school to find out the details of her behaviour there. This Mrs Brown grants. He also asks to see Annie again, in one week, this time with Mr Brown too.

In the meantime, without asking Mrs Brown's permission, he discusses the case and divulges his suspicions to an older colleague in the practice who advises him to continue to monitor the situation closely and reminds him that Annie's younger sister, Jane, could also be at risk. In terms of the Algorithm Dr Munro has progressed only as far as the third box of the External Considerations segment, where he is required to make a provisional assessment of the problem.

At the next interview, Dr Munro discovers that Annie's uncharacteristic behaviour has continued, which has been confirmed by the school. Mrs Brown is again accompanying her daughter but Mr Brown could not come because he was attending an important meeting at work. Dr Munro has become very worried about Annie's well-being, and, once alone with the mother, tentatively suggests that some form of CSA may have occurred. Taken aback, Mrs Brown firmly denies the possibility. Gently Dr Munro puts it to her that since she is not always with her daughter she cannot be certain that no-one is interfering with Annie. He says that in his opinion the safest next step would be to contact the Social Services Department. Mrs Brown says she will not allow this, in any circumstances.

Because of the disagreement Dr Munro is forced to consider his Moral Duties. He is intuitively attracted to the idea of **minimising harm**. He appreciates that to take this course means that he will have to disregard confidentiality and promise-keeping, but he believes that Mrs Brown's intransigence makes such a step necessary. Thus he contacts Social Services.

This has become a most uncomfortable case for the doctor. Although he has made his decision and acted on it after considering only two segments of the Algorithm, he decides to continue working through the instrument in order to reassure himself, and to bolster his confidence. He has a slight worry that this process might reveal a flaw in his policy, but he is prepared to take this risk, and to change his mind if he has to.

Relaxed at home, Dr Munro moves on in the Algorithm to consider the Consequences. With which category ought he to be most concerned: Annie (the individual), the Brown family (the group), himself, or wider society? Each seems important in its own way, but he knows from experience that it's unlikely that he will be able to select them all and retain harmony. He does not think that his own benefit is central in this case. Not to do anything and wait to see if things blow over might be his easiest option – one which would minimise unpleasant personal consequences – but more important factors override this consideration. Dr Munro recognises that if abuse is discovered then the family unit may disintegrate (assuming that Mr Brown is the abuser – which is by no means certain), and that even if no evidence of abuse is found the resulting stigma of the investigation may leave lasting wounds within a respectable family's life. However, it must be young Annie who is the priority. The effects on her life could be devastating.

Dr Munro next checks the Central Conditions of Health Work segment, and once again is reassured. In one sense, in each segment, he repeats his basic analysis: Annie's safety is paramount, therefore he must break confidentiality in order to ensure it. However, he need not necessarily remain convinced. Within this segment he sees a basic clash between the boxes **create autonomy** and **respect autonomy**. However, if he persists with the individual (Annie) as his priority this conflict is easily resolved. Although he is not respecting the autonomy of Mr and Mrs Brown, his action is done with the genuine intent of creating autonomy for Annie – and perhaps ultimately for the family as a whole – although this is in some doubt.

Dr Munro remains satisfied with his decision.

EXERCISE

Although the doctor is satisfied, you may not be. Some might say that Dr Munro's deliberation has been static and inflexible, and that he made up his mind without completing his ethical deliberation, and without giving alternative strategies a full airing.

Use the Algorithm to re-think the situation for Dr Munro. Bear in mind that at this stage there is no physical evidence of abuse. Has the doctor jumped the gun? Has he sacrificed a family's happiness by over-reacting? Is it the doctor's sole professional obligation to inform Social Services, or does he have greater duties? Should confidentiality be overridden so lightly? How might further investigations have been made without drawing attention to the Browns?

There are many issues to be explored in cases of suspected child abuse. Use the Algorithm imaginatively to explore alternative policies which might create a *higher degree of morality*. If necessary add further factual details to give more breadth to your analysis.

Reference

1. The Butler Schloss Report – Lord E. (1988) *Enquiry into Child Sexual Abuse in Cleveland*. London: HMSO.

Case 14

A Most Common Dilemma

Introduction

One of the most frequent misperceptions about ethics is that moral problems only occur from time to time. In fact every single medical and health care intervention is potentially morally problematic. The following case describes and discusses arguably the most common dilemma which faces GPs. The issues are presented in the format of a fourth year tutorial session on ethical issues in general practice. Ten students are present. The session is an amalgam of several real life discussions between medical undergraduates and their ethics tutor.

To Prescribe or Not?

TUTOR: Well, you've had two and a half weeks' experience observing general practice now. You've fed back on your first impressions, discussed some specific clinical issues, and considered the implications of 'informatics' for GPs. In this session I'm going to ask you to raise any ethical issues you've encountered. You should have completed Sheet V of your handbook during your practice experience. This will help you feed back. You shouldn't have had any difficulty in identifying ethical questions, not now that all fourth years take a full week ethics teaching block in September. Am I correct in this assumption, or did you have problems spotting the ethics?

JAMES: No, not at all. Most of us didn't know which issue to choose, there were so many.

TUTOR: Good. That's the thing about ethics, once you learn what ethical analysis involves . . . So, you've all got one key ethical issue to raise for discussion, and I wouldn't be surprised if some have caused you anxiety. But, before I go round the group, I wonder have any of you detected any *recurring* ethical issues? Ethical analysis is required daily of GPs (even if they don't always realise that this is what they are doing). You're lucky in having had formal tuition in ethics, which should help you make better decisions. Did anyone observe any daily dilemmas which you think we might be able to analyse with benefit?

LINDA: I have, or at least I think it's an ethical issue.

TUTOR: Good. It almost certainly will be, what did you discover?

LINDA:	Well, it's to do with prescribing antibiotics. After a few days with my GP I noticed that she was prescribing a lot of antibiotics. I began to think about whether she was doing the right thing, because it seemed to me that a lot of the patients had a viral illness.
TUTOR:	That's very interesting. Students often raise this question, and it's very important. Did you discuss it with the GP?
LINDA:	Not really. She was a bit bossy and I didn't feel right asking questions that she might think were critical of her.
BRIAN:	I felt the same with mine.
TUTOR:	This is common too. You should ask as many questions as you can, and you shouldn't be afraid. We learn through asking questions.
JOHN:	It's not as easy as you might think with some doctors.
TUTOR:	I know, but you should try anyway . . . Okay, you didn't discuss your GPs' prescription habits, but nevertheless you felt that her policy wasn't the best – do you remember that another way of saying this is to say: the policy didn't *create the highest degree of morality*? Good. Right – why not?
LINDA:	Well it was just so routine. It made the consultations very quick. I timed one at 2 minutes 15 seconds! But I thought, how boring . . . we learn all this medicine and then fill in prescription pads all day.
TUTOR:	Part of the time, yes. Perhaps general practice won't be for you . . . Could you tell us about a specific case which bothered you?
LINDA:	I can't remember one person completely accurately, but what would happen would be that someone would come in with a heavy cold and a sore throat. The doctor would ask how long it had gone on for, and if it was more than a couple of days would say something like, 'It's probably just a heavy cold, but I'll give you a prescription just to be on the safe side.' Then she'd prescribe Amoxil. I don't think she used anything else while I was there.
TUTOR:	Right, now what's wrong with that? Anybody can chip in if you like. What I'll do, whenever I can, will be to explain which bit of the Ethical Grid you are considering. Does everybody remember the Ethical Grid?
STUDENTS:	How could we forget the Ethical Grid?!
TUTOR:	Hmm . . . I don't think I'll respond to that right now!
LINDA:	I remember the Grid. Isn't the red bit to do with consequences?
TUTOR:	The green bit.
LINDA:	Yes, well I think there's a lot to do with consequences here.
TUTOR:	Go on.
LINDA:	I find it hard to see the **benefit**. It's very probable that the patients had a cold or flu virus, in which case antibiotics are useless. The only benefit I can see is that patients will feel reassured because something is being done for them.
TUTOR:	Good. You are definitely within the green layer of the Grid. Can you think of any other costs or disadvantages?
DENNIS:	There's the money. How much does Amoxil cost?
RAMESH:	I think it's about £5 for one week's course.
LINDA:	Also there can be side-effects can't there? We learnt in hospital that antibiotics stick in the dust and that eventually some bacteria learn to become resistant: 'super-bugs'! Presumably the same thing could happen in any community if antibiotics are prescribed very freely?

TUTOR:	I'm not certain. It must be a possibility though. Any other consequences?
BRIAN:	Allergic reaction. A lot of people are allergic to penicillin, for instance. It's always on their records.
CHRIS:	Imbalance of bacteria in the gut . . . diarrhoea's a possibility . . .
TUTOR:	So there's a lot to think about in terms of outcome . . . Thinking about what the Grid actually says in a green box – **most beneficial outcome for the patient** – what possible advantages can you think of ?
RAMESH:	I can think of two benefits. Patients expect doctors to be able to help them so giving antibiotics is a sort of public relations thing. The other is that the doctor doesn't know for sure that the patient has a virus, it might be bacterial. If the patient wants the doctor to do something, and it is bacterial, then giving antibiotics will be the **most beneficial outcome for the patient**.
TUTOR:	Anything else?
RAMESH:	Ummm . . . yes. You could say that if the doctor doesn't know for sure then he shouldn't take chances, and he should test . . . take a swab and a blood count. But this has consequences too. There's a wait of about five days for the results. Oh, and of course the doctor will have to see the patient again, not just once, and surgeries are crowded as it is. And there's the money cost again. The labs reckon that these sort of tests cost around £10 at the moment.
TUTOR:	So to test to make sure of infection is twice as expensive as simply prescribing the Amoxil.
LINDA:	And not to prescribe anything is free!
TUTOR:	Possibly. We seem to be focusing on negatives again. What about the two positive points that Ramesh made. Public relations and it might be beneficial?
EILEEN:	Are we still in the green level?
TUTOR:	Yes, and we've also visited the black layer from time to time. We've considered **resources available, the risk** and **the degree of certainty of the evidence**.
EILEEN:	Well, I want to be negative again. I think we should be in the green layer and looking at **benefit for society** here. Somebody mentioned crowded waiting rooms, and we've also heard about patient expectations, so there's a link here. If doctors prescribed less antibiotics then most people would recover naturally, and, since they'd get used to not visiting the surgery, workload would be reduced.
TUTOR:	Increase in benefit for oneself – the doctor?

EILEEN: Yes, and the rest of the practice, and the other patients with more serious illnesses.

TUTOR: I can see I have to be the devil's advocate here. What do you think to this: there's a 1 in 100 chance that the heavy cold and sore throat is going to get worse without antibiotics – and we can't tell with which patient; some may even develop life-threatening pneumonia. For some, antibiotics might make a really big difference. Can't we select a few boxes here to justify blanket prescribing, in the sort of conditions Eileen has described? What about **the risk, respect autonomy, most beneficial outcome for the individual patient**, and **minimise harm** (as a basic medical duty)? Isn't this safety first policy really the most moral possible?

LINDA: I don't think it is, if you don't mind me saying so. I've thought about it a lot during my practice experience, and now you've reminded us about the Grid I think I'd choose some different boxes. What nobody's mentioned yet is the blue box **create autonomy**, but I think this is the most important. What really bothered me about my GP was that she didn't take the time to talk to the patients, she didn't really explain anything, and some of them didn't even realise they'd been given antibiotics. So they didn't have much control, did they, and autonomy is about control, isn't it?

TUTOR: Yes. An autonomous person has control over his life.

LINDA: Yes, so I think doctors should tell the patients what we've been discussing – that there are **risks**, that it's not certain that antibiotics can do any good at all for their illness. I think that the costs should be mentioned too. I mean the money side of it. I think this would **create autonomy** in people and so be **the most beneficial outcome for the patient**. Also, what the doctor should do then should be to look at the box **respect autonomy** too. I think the best solution would be for the doctor, after discussion, to write out a prescription for Amoxil – whatever else – hand it to the patient but say to wait two or three days and then, if the patient's not any better, to go to the chemist. That really gives choice.

TUTOR: Good. That seems to be an excellent policy. I honestly can't see too much wrong with that. Can anybody else . . .?

EXERCISE

It is January and you are a GP faced with an epidemic of cold and flu symptoms. Your surgery resources are stretched to the limit, particularly your own time. Bearing in mind that it's far quicker to give antibiotics than an explanation, consider your policy during this busy period with the help of the Ethical Grid, or the Algorithm if you prefer.

Case 15

Allocating Resources

Introduction

The question of how to allocate available resources in a just and rational way presents apparently intractable difficulties for all health services. In some European countries (such as Sweden) governments spend as much as 10% of their gross national product (GNP) on health care[1] – and still it is not enough. This has led some observers to conclude that there is a potentially infinite demand on health care resources. They argue that as medical technology advances it will be able to meet an increasing number of 'health needs' which will in turn further fuel demand. Not everybody accepts this argument.[2] However, even if it is held that there is a limit to the funding required by a health service it is a simple fact that some resource problems occur as a result of natural scarcity. For example, there are only a limited number of surgeons with the training and talent to perform extensive heart surgery, and there is always a limit to the number of donor organs available for transplant at any given moment.

Where resources are scarce then difficult decisions have to be made by those with the power of distribution. Such decisions are not always stark and direct – should I treat Mrs Smith or Mrs Jones – but may be made at levels apparently quite removed from wards and surgeries. Nevertheless, each decision to allocate a valued resource to one place rather than another is of ethical concern.

The following case reveals something of the reality and complexity of decision making in health care where resources are scarce, and serves also as a reminder of a question for doctors first raised in Case 4: *do I have an obligation to my patient only, or do I have obligations to others not directly in my care? And if I do have obligations, do these obligations ever outweigh those I have to my patient?*

What is Fair?

The situation

Melchester Health Authority (MHA) was placed in a position where it had to reduce its expenditure in order to achieve a balanced budget. The Department of Health provided an 'overall cash limited' increase of 8.3% as follows:

1990/91 inflation provision	5.0%
General growth provision	2.5%
Earmarked growth provision	0.8%
TOTAL	8.3%

The budgeting review indicated that MHA faced a recurring deficit of £443,000. Consequently several cuts had to be made, particularly to community health services. A new post was established for a consultant paediatrician (in keeping with national guidelines) while six other jobs were lost, including three school nurses and an administrator in the Geriatric Department. Several family planning clinics were closed – it was argued that GPs could and should take on this responsibility.

Your task

Unlike all but one other case in this book, this example is not analysed with use of the Grid or the Algorithm. Following its presentation advice is given, but the onus is on the reader of the case (or the group discussing the case) to go through the necessary steps independently. Of course, if it is decided to use the Algorithm the procedure is predetermined.

The problem to be analysed

MHA has contacted you for whatever advice you can offer over its general procedures for resource allocation, with particular reference to the following case.

John is 23 years old. He had a road accident in March 1988 and suffered severe head injuries. He was a student of computing at Oxford University at the time of his accident. After he recovered from his initial injuries John was able to communicate simple needs, but had significant speech problems. Later he became able to walk around normally, to feed himself and to paint – but had frequent memory lapses. Every few minutes he would find himself in a room, not knowing why he was there, not recognise the room, and not be able to return to his starting point.

The consultant at the local hospital argued that the Health Authority should pay for John to undergo rehabilitative treatment at a private hospital in Easthampton. His parents, who had been looking after him for the previous four years, were strongly in favour of this, not least for the respite it would give them. There are, however, several schools of thought regarding the effectiveness of the treatment methods used by the private unit. You should also take account of the fact that the consultant had been pushing for a local unit for people with severe spine and head injuries, and a bid had been made to the Regional Health Authority for funding.

In other words, you will need to pay close attention to both the red and green levels of the decision-making implements. You will need to consider carefully the motives of the protagonists as well as the actual and potential outcomes of the decisions taken.

The Health Authority agreed to fund John's care in the private hospital for six months at a cost of £26,000. At the same time it agreed that seven other patients with problems like John's should receive private rehabilitative care. The total cost was approximately £300,000 per annum.

After six months John's case was reviewed. He had made very slow progress, but the Team at the rehabilitation centre advised that the benefits of the six months' therapy would soon start to show. The Health Authority agreed to fund John's placement for a further six months until December 1991. But in the meantime the Health Authority closed a surgical ward and stopped all routine surgery for three months because of an overspend on its budget. Cuts in the preceding six months had also occurred in Community Health Services.

In December a case conference was held. The local consultant advised that John should remain at the private hospital – pointing out again what a strong case the District had for the Regional Health Authority to fund a local unit. John's keyworker considered that he was unlikely to make any substantial progress and that he should return to the community to live with his parents with back up from social and health services. The Unit General Manager finally concluded that it was necessary to withdraw John's funding, and John returned to his parents within a week.

A few days later, solicitors acting for John's parents wrote to the local MP complaining that funding for John's care had arbitrarily been withdrawn by the Health Authority. They asked that the matter be taken up by the Health Minister.

John is now a client of the Social Services Department of the London Borough of Melchester. The long-term plan is to find him a home which is suited to his needs, and where he will mix with people of his own age. John attends the Broomhall Day Centre in Edgebury for three days per week and has the option to attend for five days if he wishes.

Advice on Analysis

As you attempt to deal with this case you will feel the need for more information. For example, what are the conditions of the people denied routine surgery? What are their incomes? What are their backgrounds? If you wish, and deem it necessary, you should fill in these details. However, in cases like this (in real life too), no matter how much information you possess you could say that you still require more to make a properly informed decision.

How long will John live for? What pleasure does he have? Is he suffering in any sense? What effect does the loss of a geriatric administrator have on the people on the ward? What are the benefits of the extra consultant paediatrician? In real-life decision making there are always inaccessible unknowns. The task is, always, to make the best and most defensible decision within the limits of knowledge.

It may be best to think of your task as one of *principle. What ought the priority of a Health Authority be, and how might such a priority be argued for in the face of alternatives? What might be the practical implications of ranking principles be?*

If you are to use the Grid to deal with this case remember that it is always necessary to ask a specific question (for example, is the consultant's policy the best possible? Should the Health Authority treat only those people with a good chance of recovery?) Then, all that is required is that each coloured layer is at least thought about. It matters little which layer is chosen as the point of entry, although in this case an obvious 'way in' is to begin in the green section in order to try to sort out some idea of (a) which outcomes are thought to be desirable, and (b) which people, or groups of people, are felt to be priorities. You might also choose to re-read the discussion of principles in the Introduction to the book.

References

1. Lindgren, B. (1989) Swedish health systems. *Health Care Financing Review Annual Supplement*, pp. 66–71.
2. Smith, A. (1987) Qualms about QALYs. *Lancet* i: 1134–6.

Conclusion

The Appeal to Reason

This book has shown that there are different ways to tackle ethical problems in medicine and health care, and has recommended two approaches which couple flexibility with systematic thinking. These methods place the initial onus of responsibility firmly on the individual who has to deal with ethically difficult situations. By insisting on comprehensive personal analysis – which must draw on a combination of principles and facts – the strategies advocated here depart from a deeply established tradition of rule-following in medicine. Although for much of the time the analyst will arrive at familiar solutions, the Grid and its derivative leave open the possibility of originality.

The problem-solving methods explained in these pages allow decision-makers to respond creatively to unique puzzles, rather than habitually be constrained by precedent. In other words the methodology of the Ethical Grid permits an ultimate *appeal to reason* rather than *appeal to authority*. This is an essential insight into the nature of ethical analysis, and the most appropriate conclusion to this casebook.

Appeals to authority

Such appeals take different forms but are primarily these:

- A doctor might follow the advice or defer to the opinion of others. For instance, his choice of response might be dictated by a senior colleague or a court of law.
- A doctor might follow policies in accord with his professional codes of practice. In other words he might look up what to do in the rule book.
- A doctor might have set procedures, which she has made use of in the past, and always follow these in situations which appear to be similar.

These appeals to authority share in common a deference to sources which are never unique to the context under examination, and which have always been specified in advance.

Appeals to reason

Appeals to reason may consider and follow authorities, but they need not necessarily do so. Instead, with this approach, each circumstance is thought through systematically in order to reach the best possible solution.

Naturally the same eventual conclusions can be reached by either *authority* or *reason*. But even though an identical answer may be reached there are hugely important differences in the other outcomes of an appeal to reason. The most significant of these are:

- That the decision-maker will understand as fully as possible the basis for his decision, whereas if he merely follows *authority* he may have only a hazy view of the justification for it.
- That the decision-maker will have grown personally as a result of rising to the ethical challenge: not only may she have learnt fresh insights and discovered alternative outlooks on the situation, but she will have genuinely confronted a problem as a person, and not sheltered behind the label 'professional'. In other words, the *appeal to reason* guarantees that the problem has personal meaning for the decision-maker because it must become *her* problem.
- That the decision-maker will be able to articulate to others the basis of her decision. With access to the Grid or Algorithm, anybody – whether doctor, nurse, manager or patient – will be able to see the point of (or to challenge) the decision in the same terms as it was made. In this way *appeal to reason* makes ethical decision-making readily accessible to public scrutiny.

One consequence of this final benefit of the *appeal to reason* is that the public at large will be more able to ask questions of a doctor's ethical analysis, but this may look to some to be a demand that doctors sacrifice authority. However this cannot be the case because doctors have never had any special authority in ethical analysis – no group of people of any description can claim superiority in this sort of decision-making: no-one has privileged knowledge of ethical truths. All that is possible is for the process to be more or less efficient, and more or less comprehensive. Prowess in moral analysis can be learnt, but requires much practice. And it is self-evident that the best reasoning can flourish only if ideas are shared, borrowed, discussed and tested in the arena of open debate.

Index

Index compiled by John Gibson